FOGSI EEBR 2025

Ethical Evidence-Based Recommendations

Fibroids

AF729911

Disclaimer

This Ethical Evidence-Based Recommendation (EEBR) document is drafted following a consensus between esteemed FOGSI experts and stakeholders and are based on the scientific evidence available at the time of preparation.

EEBRs should be used for information and educational purposes. They do not replace the need for application of clinical judgment to each individual presentation, or variations based on individual patient and resource setting.

Furthermore, EEBRs do not constitute or imply the endorsement of any of the included technologies, therapies, or techniques by FOGSI.

FOGSI EEBR 2025

Ethical Evidence-Based Recommendations

Fibroids

Editor-in-Chief

Sunita Tandulwadkar

MD (Obs and Gyne) FICS (Gyne-Endoscopy) FICOG
President, FOGSI (2025–2026)
Gynecological Endoscopist and ART & IVF Specialist
Head, Department of Obstetrics and Gynecology
Chief, IVF & Endoscopy Center, Ruby Hall Clinic, Pune
Founder and Medical Director
Solo Clinic IVF—A Center for Excellence in Infertility and Endoscopy, Pune
Founder and Medical Director
Solo Stem Cells—A Stem Cell Research and Application Center, Pune
Founder and Director, Alive Regenerative Wellness, Pune, Maharashtra, India

Editors

Basab Mukherjee

MD FRCOG FICOG
Consultant
Department of Obstetrics and Gynecology
Ankuran Fertility and Fetal Medicine Center
Kolkata, West Bengal, India

Soumil Trivedi

DNB FMIGS FICOG
Co-Director and Consultant
Department of Obstetrics and Gynecology
Dr Trivedi's Total Health Care and
AAKAR IVF Centre
Mumbai, Maharashtra, India

Experts

Aswath Kumar

MD FICOG
Professor
Department of Gynecology
Jubilee Mission Medical College
Thrissur, Kerala, India

Subhash Mallya

DNB DGO MNAMS FICOG Diploma in
Gynec Endoscopy (Germany)
Senior Consultant and Head
Department of Minimal Access Gynecology
Baby memorial Hospital
Kozhikode, Kerala, India

Convener

Pooja Lodha

DNB (Obs and Gyne)
Fellow, Fetal Medicine, FOGSI-FMF UK Certified
Lead Consultant
Department of Fetal Medicine
Ruby Hall Clinic and Bharati Vidyapeeth University and Hospital, Pune
Director, Kangaroo Cradle, Fetal Care Centre
Pune, Maharashtra, India

JAYPEE BROTHERS MEDICAL PUBLISHERS

The Health Sciences Publisher

New Delhi | London

JAYPEE **Jaypee Brothers Medical Publishers (P) Ltd**

Headquarters
Jaypee Brothers Medical Publishers (P) Ltd
EMCA House, 23/23-B
Ansari Road, Daryaganj
New Delhi 110 002, India
Landline: +91-11-23272143, +91-11-23272703
+91-11-23282021, +91-11-23245672
Email: jaypee@jaypeebrothers.com

Corporate Office
Jaypee Brothers Medical Publishers (P) Ltd
4838/24, Ansari Road, Daryaganj
New Delhi 110 002, India
Phone: +91-11-43574357
Fax: +91-11-43574314
Email: jaypee@jaypeebrothers.com

Overseas Office
JP Medical Ltd.
83, Victoria Street, London
SW1H 0HW (UK)
Phone: +44 20 3170 8910
Fax: +44 (0)20 3008 6180
Email: info@jpmedpub.com

Website: www.jaypeebrothers.com
Website: www.jaypeedigital.com

© 2025, Jaypee Brothers Medical Publishers

The views and opinions expressed in this book are solely those of the original contributor(s)/author(s) and do not necessarily represent those of editor(s) or publisher of the book.

All rights reserved. No part of this publication may be reproduced, stored or transmitted in any form or by any means, electronic, mechanical, photocopying, recording or otherwise, without the prior permission in writing of the publishers.

All brand names and product names used in this book are trade names, service marks, trademarks or registered trademarks of their respective owners. The publisher is not associated with any product or vendor mentioned in this book.

Medical knowledge and practice change constantly. This book is designed to provide accurate, authoritative information about the subject matter in question. However, readers are advised to check the most current information available on procedures included and check information from the manufacturer of each product to be administered, to verify the recommended dose, formula, method and duration of administration, adverse effects and contraindications. It is the responsibility of the practitioner to take all appropriate safety precautions. Neither the publisher nor the author(s)/editor(s) assume any liability for any injury and/or damage to persons or property arising from or related to use of material in this book.

This book is sold on the understanding that the publisher is not engaged in providing professional medical services. If such advice or services are required, the services of a competent medical professional should be sought.

Every effort has been made where necessary to contact holders of copyright to obtain permission to reproduce copyright material. If any have been inadvertently overlooked, the publisher will be pleased to make the necessary arrangements at the first opportunity.

Inquiries for bulk sales may be solicited at: jaypee@jaypeebrothers.com

FOGSI EEBR 2025—Ethical Evidence-Based Recommendations: Fibroids

First Edition: **2025**

ISBN: 978-93-6616-245-4

Printed in India

Contributors

Alok Sharma
MD MICOG FICOG DHA
Consultant
Department of Obstetrics and Gynecology
Civil Hospital
Mandi, Himachal Pradesh, India

Amrutha Pentakota
MS (Obs and Gyne) Fellow in MAS
Former Assistant Professor
Vydehi Institute of Medical Sciences
Bengaluru, Karnataka, India
Department of Obstetrics and Gynecology
Apollo Hospitals
Hyderabad, Telangana, India

Anahita Chauhan
MD DGO DFP FICOG
Consultant and Head
Department of Obstetrics and Gynecology
Saifee Hospital
Mumbai, Maharashtra, India

Annith Kumar VM
MS (Obs and Gyne) MRCOG
Scientific Director
Promise Fertility Center, Chennai
Assistant Professor
Department of Obstetrics and Gynecology
Tagore Medical College
Chennai, Tamil Nadu, India

Anupama Dave
MS DNB MRCOG FACOG FICS
Professor and Unit Head
Department of Obstetrics and Gynecology
MGM Medical College and MTH Hospital
Indore, Madhya Pradesh, India

Aswath Kumar
MD FICOG
Professor
Department of Gynecology
Jubilee Mission Medical College
Thrissur, Kerala, India

Basab Mukherjee
MD FRCOG FICOG
Consultant
Department of Obstetrics and Gynecology
Ankuran Fertility and Fetal Medicine Center
Kolkata, West Bengal, India

Bidisha Roychoudhury
DNB (Obs and Gyne) MRCOG FMAS FIAOG
Assistant Professor
Department of Obstetrics and Gynecology
Institute of Post Graduate Medical Education and Research
Kolkata, West Bengal, India

Charu Mittal
MD DNB MICOG MNAMS
Consultant
Department of Obstetrics and Gynecology
Nidaan Hospital
Gwalior, Madhya Pradesh, India

Himleena Gautam
MS DNB FMAS
Consultant
Department of Obstetrics and Gynecology
Apollo Hospitals
Guwahati, Assam, India

Kaustav Kar
MBBS (Hons) MS (Obs and Gyne) FRM FMIGS
Consultant Obstetrician, Gynecologist and Infertility Specialist
Department of Obstetrics and Gynecology
Mediland Hospital and Research Centre
Silchar, Assam, India

Monika Anant
MBBS MS FICOG FMAS
Professor
Department of Obstetrics and Gynecology
All India Institute of Medical Sciences
Patna, Bihar, India

Munjal Pandya
MS (Obs and Gyne) FICOG DMIS
Associate Professor
Department of Obstetrics and Gynecology
Narendra Modi Medical College
Ahmedabad, Gujarat, India

Poushali Sanyal
MS DNB MRCOG FMAS
Consultant
Department of Obstetrics and Gynecology
Woodlands Hospital
Kolkata, West Bengal, India

Prakash Trivedi
MD DNB DGO FCPS FICOG
Director and Head
Department of Obstetrics and Gynecology
Dr Trivedi's Total Health Care and AAKAR IVF Centre
Mumbai, Maharashtra, India

Ramprasad Dey
MD DCH FICOG FMAS
Professor
Department of Obstetrics and Gynecology
Medical College
Kolkata, West Bengal, India

Rashmika Gandhi
MBBS MS (Obs and Gyne) DNB FRM
Fellowship in Gyne Endoscopy
Associate Consultant
Department of Fertility and IVF
Birla Fertility and IVF
Gurugram, Haryana, India

Rooma Sinha MD (Obs and Gyne)
Clinical Lead
Robotic Gynecological Surgery
Department of Gynecology
Apollo Hospitals
Hyderabad, Telangana, India

S Krishnakumar MS (Obs and Gyne)
Laparoscopic Surgeon, Infertility Specialist
Department of Obstetrics and Gynecology
JK Women Hospital
Dombivli, Maharashtra, India

Sanket Pisat MBBS MS DNB FICOG
Consultant Gynecological Endoscopic Surgeon
Department of Obstetrics and Gynecology
Akanksha Womens Hospital
Mumbai, Maharashtra, India

Sejal Naik
MS (Obs and Gyne) FMAS FRM FICOG
Director and Consultant
Department of Obstetrics and Gynecology
Belly and Love Women's Care
Surat, Gujarat, India

Shehla Jamal
MBBS DNB
Professor and Unit Head
Department of Obstetrics and Gynecology, Medical Education
Rajshree Medical Research Institute
Bareilly, Uttar Pradesh, India

Shobha N Gudi
MD DNB FICOG CIMP FKCOG
Professor and Head
Department of Obstetrics and Gynecology
St Philomena's Hospital
Bengaluru, Karnataka, India

Shrutika O Makde
MS (Obs and Gyne) DNB (Obs and Gyne)
Assistant Professor
Department of Obstetrics and Gynecology
Lokmanya Tilak Municipal Medical College and Government Hospital
Mumbai, Maharashtra, India

Soumil Trivedi DNB FMIGS FICOG
Co-Director and Consultant
Department of Obstetrics and Gynecology
Dr Trivedi's Total Health Care and AAKAR IVF Centre
Mumbai, Maharashtra, India

Subhash Mallya
DNB DGO MNAMS FICOG Diploma in Gynec Endoscopy (Germany)
Senior Consultant and Head
Department of Minimal Access Gynecology
Baby memorial Hospital
Kozhikode, Kerala, India

Suchita Pisat MBBS DGO FICOG
Consultant Gynecologist
Department of Obstetrics and Gynecology
Akanksha Womens Hospital
Mumbai, Maharashtra, India

Sunita Tandulwadkar
MD (Obs and Gyne) FICS (Gyne-Endoscopy) FICOG
President, FOGSI (2025–2026)
Gynecological Endoscopist and ART & IVF Specialist
Head, Department of Obstetrics and Gynecology
Chief, IVF & Endoscopy Center
Ruby Hall Clinic, Pune
Founder and Medical Director
Solo Clinic IVF—A Center for Excellence in Infertility and Endoscopy, Pune
Founder and Medical Director
Solo Stem Cells—A Stem Cell Research and Application Center, Pune
Founder and Director
Alive Regenerative Wellness
Pune, Maharashtra, India

Suyash Naval
DNB FAGLS Bachelor in Endoscopy (ESGE)
Consultant
Department of Obstetrics and Gynecology
Naval Multi Specialty Hospital
Jalgaon, Maharashtra, India

Tulika Jha DGO MS FICOG
Associate Professor
Department of Obstetrics and Gynecology
Raiganj Government Medical College and Hospital
Kolkata, West Bengal, India

Vatsla Vats
MBBS MS DNB (Obs and Gyne) Fellowship in Minimal Access Surgery, Trained in Reproductive Medicine
Associate Consultant
Department of Obstetrics and Gynecology
Motherhood
Gurugram, Haryana, India

Venugopal M MD DNB
Consultant and Center Head
Department of Reproductive Medicine
Birla ARMC IVF
Thrissur, Kerala, India

Preface

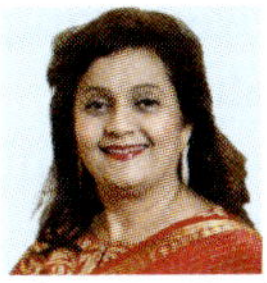

Editor-in-Chief
Sunita Tandulwadkar

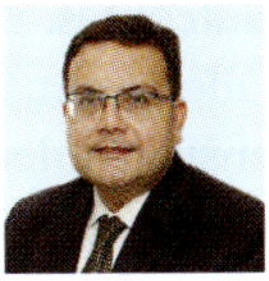

Editor
Basab Mukherjee

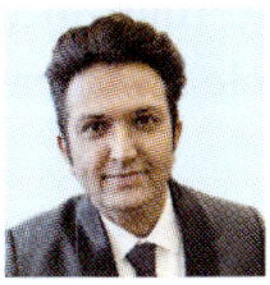

Editor
Soumil Trivedi

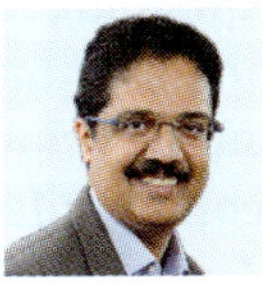

Expert
Aswath Kumar

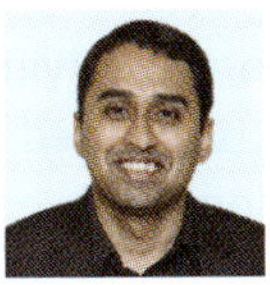

Expert
Subhash Mallya

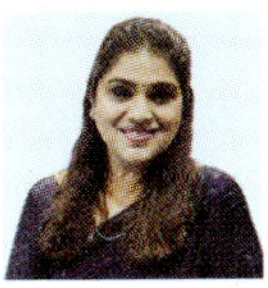

Convener
Pooja Lodha

In our pursuit of advancing women's health in India, establishing our own ethical evidence-based recommendations is essential. As President of the Federation of Obstetric and Gynaecological Societies of India (FOGSI) 2025, I am delighted to present this *Ethical Evidence-Based Recommendations on Fibroids*, a comprehensive resource developed through the collective expertise of leading professionals across the country. While international bodies such the International Federation of Gynecology and Obstetrics (FIGO), American Society for Reproductive Medicine (ASRM), European Society of Human Reproduction and Embryology (ESHRE), and Royal College of Obstetricians and Gynaecologists (RCOG) have established extensive recommendations, India has yet to provide a consolidated, evidence-backed framework for fibroids. This publication bridges that gap, providing Indian practitioners with a practical and thorough set of recommendations for diagnosing and managing fibroids in various clinical contexts.

Fibroids, or myomas, are complex benign tumors with diverse presentations, influencing a wide spectrum of women's health outcomes. These ethical evidence-based recommendations begin by detailing the origins, etiology, pathophysiology, and risk factors associated with fibroids, giving practitioners a foundational understanding of hormonal, genetic, and environmental influences. Further, the clinical presentation and various fibroid locations are explored, including atypical fibroids and degeneration patterns, to help practitioners recognize and manage diverse fibroid manifestations effectively.

A dedicated section addresses the impact of myomas on fertility, detailing approaches for managing fibroids in women seeking conception. It covers the prevalence of fibroids in infertility cases, their effect on fertility outcomes, and options for both surgical and nonsurgical management to support fertility, including insights for assisted reproductive technology (ART) scenarios. Diagnostic modalities, including ultrasound and magnetic resonance imaging (MRI), and the role of hormonal assays are thoroughly reviewed, equipping practitioners with evidence-backed protocols for fibroid evaluation.

Management recommendations extend to asymptomatic fibroids, considering the age-specific needs of adolescent, reproductive, and perimenopausal women. The publication also addresses the intersection of fibroids and pregnancy, highlighting implications for both mother and fetus and providing management strategies that ensure optimal outcomes.

Both medical and surgical management options are detailed extensively. Medical approaches cover options for managing heavy menstrual bleeding and emerging therapies, while surgical recommendations span various myomectomy techniques, including open, laparoscopic, hysteroscopic, robotic, and innovative methods like vNOTES. Additionally, alternative modalities such as uterine artery embolization (UAE) and high-intensity focused ultrasound (HIFU) offer noninvasive choices, with clear indications, contraindications, and fertility considerations.

The publication also includes recommendations on the risk of malignancy, psychological, and medicolegal implications of fibroids, recognizing the holistic impact of fibroid management on patient care.

This publication represents FOGSI's commitment to equipping Indian gynecologists with the latest scientific advancements, framed within our cultural and clinical context. I am deeply grateful to the multidisciplinary team whose collaborative efforts have made these recommendations possible. We hope that they become a trusted companion for practitioners, empowering them to deliver compassionate, evidence-based care for patients with fibroids.

Through this initiative, FOGSI reaffirms its dedication to advancing women's health and setting a new standard for ethical, informed care. We trust that these ethical evidence-based recommendations will serve as both a valuable guide and an inspiration for the management of fibroids across India.

Contents

CHAPTER 1

Origin, Etiology, Pathophysiology, Epidemiology, and Risk Factors of Uterine Fibroids

Ramprasad Dey, Himleena Gautam

INTRODUCTION

Uterine fibroids are one of the most common benign pelvic neoplasms in women, mostly found in the reproductive age group. It is a smooth muscle tumor with fibrous connective tissue. Around 70% of women may develop fibroids. They are a cause of significant morbidity and is considered the most common cause of hysterectomy worldwide, posing a significant health and financial burden.

Q1. What is the origin of fibroids and what are the molecular and genetic mechanisms underlying its development?

- Genetic transformation of a myometrial stem cell to tumor initiating cell (TIC) leads to development of fibroids.
- Various genetic and chromosomal alterations lead to monoclonal expansion of the TIC, the most common being MED12 mutations.
- Myofibroblasts produce extracellular matrix (ECM) which further promotes growth of fibroids
- Various growth factors and cytokines are implicated in fibroid growth

Summary of evidence: A genetic hit is the first step in pathogenesis of fibroids. Myometrial stem cells, present in normal myometrium, undergo various mutations, probably because of uterine hypoxia, aberrant methylation, abnormal estrogen signaling and increased steroid hormones and transform to fibroid progenitor cells/tumor initiating cells (TIC). A single TIC then multiplies to form a myoma. Thus, fibroids are clonal in origin; but in a uterus, different fibroids arise from different TICs, each having differential gene expressions, thus maintaining heterogeneity. The most common genetic mutations include somatic mutations in mediator complex subunit 12 (MED12) gene, found in nearly 45–90% of myomas, followed by chromosomal rearrangements in high mobility group AT-hook 2 (HMGA2) seen in 7.5–10% of fibroids.

Myofibroblasts derived from smooth muscle cells, fibroblasts or somatic stem cells, are activated by inflammation, hypoxia, oxidative stress and tissue injury, and they proliferate, produce and remodel extracellular matrix (ECM).

The genetic and epigenetic mutations and chromosomal aberrations affect different receptor pathways and cellular processes causing release of growth factors, cytokines and chemokines from myocytes and ECM, which target the cells for fibroid growth.

Q2. How does hormones influence pathogenesis of uterine fibroids?

- Higher estrogen and progesterone receptors are found in fibroids
- Progesterone is the main hormone causing fibroid growth
- Exogeneous hormones like COCs and DMPA are not shown to increase fibroid growth and may have a protective effect

Summary of evidence: Studies have shown higher estrogen (OGN) and progesterone (PGN) receptors in the leiomyomas than surrounding myometrium. Estrogen regulates genes expression and promotes progesterone receptor expression. Fibroids also produce OGN locally through aromatase enzyme, which is found in myomas. PGN is the main hormone implicated in fibroid growth. It induces cell proliferation, suppresses apoptosis, produces growth factors, regulates cytokines, promotes angiogenesis and remodels ECM. High serum levels of OGN and PGN are associated with higher risk of fibroids.

Though there is a theoretical risk of increased risk when using exogenous hormones. However various studies have shown protective effect of long-term use of COCs on development of fibroids. Some studies have shown conflicting results. Use of COCs or progesterone like DMPA used to control heavy menstrual bleeding in fibroids have not shown to increase fibroid size. However, monitoring is advised. Further large population studies are needed to provide high quality evidence.

Q3. What is the natural history of fibroids?

- Fibroids are most common in reproductive age group (30–50 years), incidence gradually increasing with age.
- Annual growth rate varies widely with some undergoing shrinkage, despite of stable hormonal environment.
- Secondary changes can occur due to ischemia, vascular insult or hormonal changes
- After menopause fibroids gradually shrink
- HRT can cause regrowth of fibroids, especially in the initial 2 years.

Summary of evidence: Fibroids have never been reported before menarche with very few cases reported in the adolescent age group. Prevalence is high in the age group of 30–50 years incidence gradually increases from 20 to 60 years. Studies report average growth rates ranging from 18–82% per year, with higher rates in more vascular tumors. Spontaneous regression seen in 7–11% fibroids. Growth rate slows down with aging. During this growth period various types of secondary changes are observed in response to various insults-hyaline, cystic, fatty, calcific or red degenerations. After menopause, the growth rate stabilizes and size of fibroids start shrinking. Use of hormone replacement therapy (HRT), may cause regrowth of the lesions, causing symptoms. Thus, these patients need routine follow up.

The changes that occur in pregnancy has been discussed in separate section.

Q4. Are there any racial or ethnic disparities in natural history of fibroids?

- Highest prevalence seen in blacks, followed by Hispanics, as compared to whites
- Genetics and environmental factors are responsible for these disparities
- Black women develop fibroids early and suffer severe symptoms
- India has a high burden of uterine fibroids

Summary of evidence: Between 18–65 years of age, Black women have higher prevalence of 18.5% compared to whites with prevalence of 10.3%. The incidence may be 3 times higher in blacks and 2 times higher in Hispanic women as compared to whites. The reasons for these differences may be differential expression of around 1470 genes and micro-RNAs as well as differences in stress levels, diet, physical activities, use of beauty products, environmental and occupational exposures between these races. Black women develop myomas at early age, have multiple numbers and higher volume and have more severe symptoms. In India, various studies have shown prevalence ranging from 4.5% to 70% in the 30–50 years age group. Various studies on the risk in Asian women have shown conflicting results, with some showing risk similar to blacks and some showing similar to Caucasians.

Q5. Are there any familial or hereditary associations of fibroids?

- There is a strong familial predisposition of fibroids
- Concordance is high in monozygotic twins compared to dizygotic twins
- Some genetic disorders are associated with familial leiomyomas like HLRCC and Alport's syndrome

Summary of evidence: Various studies have shown a familial predisposition of fibroids, with risk ranging from 8–70%. Risk of developing myomas can be up to 2.5 times higher in first degree relatives of women having myomas. Also, fibroids can be almost 2 times more in monozygotic twins as compared to dizygotic twins. Some rare familial genetic disorders are also associated with fibroids. Hereditary leiomyomatosis and renal cell carcinoma (HLRCC), an autosomal dominant syndrome, involving the fumarate hydratase (FH) gene, is characterized by both cutaneous and uterine fibroids. Another hereditary disorder of type IV collagen is the Alport syndrome, caused by COL4A5, COL4A6 mutations, where there is associated nephropathy, deafness, ocular abnormalities and diffuse leiomyomatosis. Other associated genetic syndromes are Reed's, Proteus and Cowden's syndromes.

Q6. What are the risk factors, apart from genetics and race, that influence development of fibroids?

- No specific etiology has been found for fibroids
- With increasing age, chances of developing fibroids significantly increase
- Early menarche and nulliparity are found to increase risk of fibroids
- Obesity, hypertension, sedentary lifestyle and high mental stress increase risk of fibroids.
- Vitamin D deficiency and high dietary fat also increases risk of fibroids.
- Exposure to EDCs and air pollution have shown positive association with fibroids.

Summary of evidence: Etiology of fibroids is unknown. However, various risk factors have been found to play role in the development of fibroids apart from racial, ethnic and genetic causes. These are:

- *Age:* Women between 41–60 years of age have 10times higher risk of developing fibroids as compared to 21–30 years of age. In African American women incidence is 60% below 45 years, which is 80% at ≥50 years. In white women, 40% of <35 years have fibroids and 70% of >50 years have fibroids.
- *Early menarche:* This leads to increased exposure to reproductive hormones causing higher mutations in genes.
- *Parity:* Nulliparous women have higher risk of developing fibroids than multiparous ones.
- *Obesity:* Higher BMI, higher waist-to-hip ratios and fat percentage of >30% increase risk of having fibroids. Postmenopausal women who are obese, have type 2 DM and those who have taken HRT have higher risk.
- *Hypertension:* Hypertension increases the risk by 5 times.
- *Dietary factors:* Green vegetables, fruits, fish and yogurt reduce risk of developing fibroids. Consumption of ham, beef have shown to increase risk, whereas consumption of dairy products has shown conflicting associations in various studies.
- *Vitamin D:* Vitamin D deficiency is strongly associated with higher risk of fibroids.
- *Lifestyle factors:* Reduced physical activity, increased stress, childhood adversity may influence fibroid risk. Alcohol, mostly beer intake is associated with fibroid risk in dose dependent manner. Caffeine intake also increases risk.

- *Environmental exposure:*
  - Endocrine-disrupting chemicals (EDCs)—these compounds that can alter functioning of the endocrine system, have positive association with fibroids. These include Bisphenol A (BPA), benzophenone-3, triclosan, triclocarban, parabens, phthalates, etc., found in various beauty products, water bottles, beverages canned foods, pesticides etc. Prenatal exposure to DES, which is an EDC, increases risk by around 2 fold.
  - Air pollution—Chronic exposure to air pollution increases risk of fibroids.
- *Oral contraceptive pills (OCPs):* Early use of OCPS at 13–16 years of age have shown positive association than those who were not exposed at that age.

BIBLIOGRAPHY

1. Baird DD, Patchel SA, Saldana TM, et al. Uterine fibroid incidence and growth in an ultrasound-based, prospective study of young African Americans. Am J Obstetr Gynecol. 2020;223(3):402.e1-402.
2. Katon JG, Plowden TC, Marsh EE. Racial disparities in uterine fibroids and endometriosis: a systematic review and application of social, structural, and political context. Fertil Steril. 2023;119(3):355-63.
3. Keizer AL, Semmler A, Kok HS, et al. Modifiable prognostic factors in uterine fibroid development: a systematic review of literature. J Obstetr Gynaecol. 2024;44(1):2288225.
4. Koltsova AS, Efimova OA, Pendina AA. A view on uterine leiomyoma genesis through the prism of genetic, epigenetic and cellular heterogeneity. Int J Mole Sci. 2023;24(6):5752.
5. Larraín D, Prado J. (2024). New Insights into Molecular Pathogenesis of Uterine Fibroids: From the Lab to a Clinician-Friendly Review. Soft Tissue Sarcoma and Leiomyoma - Diagnosis, Management, and New Perspectives. [online] Available from http://dx.doi.org/10.5772/intechopen.1002969 [Last accessed November, 2024].
6. Lin CY, Wang CM, Chen ML, et al. The effects of exposure to air pollution on the development of uterine fibroids. Int J Hygiene Environm Health. 2019;222(3):549-55.
7. Ngorili GS, Yadav BB, Takalkar AA. Epidemiological study of uterine fibroids: Our experience from urban Maharashtra. Int J Reprod Contr Obstetr Gynecol. 2022;11(8):2101.
8. Sembene PM, Keneme B. Epidemiology and Genetic Molecular Mechanisms involved in Fibroids. Cohesive J Microbiol Infect Dis. 2021;5(3).
9. Stewart EA, Cookson CL, Gandolfo RA, et al. Epidemiology of Uterine Fibroids: A Systematic Review. BJOG. 2017;124(10):1501-12.
10. Ulin M, Ali M, Chaudhry ZT, et al. Uterine fibroids in menopause and perimenopause. Menopause (New York, N.Y.). 2020;27(2):238-42.

11. Wong JY, Gold EB, Johnson WO, et al. Circulating Sex Hormones and Risk of Uterine Fibroids: Study of Women's Health Across the Nation (SWAN). J Clin Endocrinol Metabol. 2016;101(1):123-30.
12. Yang Q, Ciebiera M, Bariani MV, et al. Comprehensive Review of Uterine Fibroids: Developmental Origin, Pathogenesis, and Treatment. Endocr Rev. 2022;43(4):678-719.

CHAPTER 2

Clinical Presentation, Different Locations including Atypical Fibroids, Various Degenerations in Fibroids

Tulika Jha, Ramprasad Dey

Q1. What are the different types of fibroids and their typical locations within the uterus?

As per position and location of fibroid in relation to uterine layers it is classified broadly as *uterine and extrauterine.*

Uterine fibroids are:

- Intramural or interstitial—most common 60%. Actually, all leiomyoma starts growing as intramural, then remains as intramural or becomes subserosal or submucosal. According FIGO classification system 3 and 4 are intramural. This type of fibroids commonly present with HMB, menorrhagia.
- Subserosal—20% (subgroup—sessile, pedunculated, parasitic, or wandering). According FIGO classification system 5, 6, and 7 are subserosal. This type of fibroids with long pedicle may have chances for torsion. Sometimes rapture of vessels from surface of subserosal fibroid may result intraperitoneal hemorrhages.
- Submucosal—20%. According FIGO classification system 0, 1, and 2 are submucosal. It may be sessile or pedunculated. Sometimes submucosal fibroid may form fibroid polyp. Intermenstrual bleeding, metrorrhagia may be a common presentation.

As per location into the uterus, it can be classified as—fundal, corporal, and cervical.

Extrauterine may arise from anywhere where there is Mullerian tissue.

Broad ligament (True or Pseudo), ovarian ligament, uterosacral, round ligament, vulva, vagina, parasitic or wandering.

FIGO leiomyoma subclassification system:

FIGO leiomyoma subclassification system

PALM	
Polyp	
Adenomyosis	**S**ubmucous
Leiomyoma	**O**ther
Malignancy and hyperplasia	

COEIN
Coagulopathy
Ovulatory dysfunction
Endometrial
Iatrogenic
Not otherwise classified

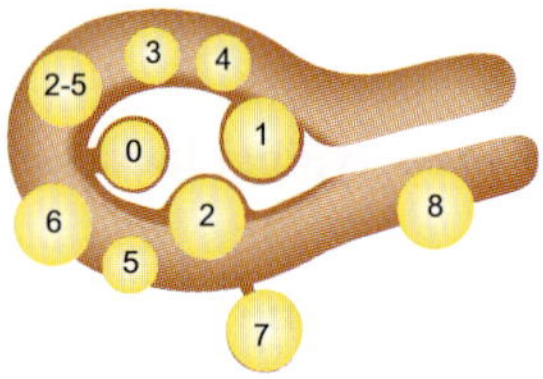

SM-Submucous	0	Pedunculated intracavitary
	1	<50% intramural
	2	≥50% intramural
	3	Contacts endometrium; 100% intramural
O-Other	4	Intramural
	5	Subserous ≥50% intramural
	6	Subserous <50% intramural
	7	Subserous pedunculated
	8	Other (specify e.g. cervical, parasitic)
Hybrid (contact both the endometrium and the serosal layer)		Two numbers are listed separated by a hyphen. By convention, the first refers to the relationship with the endometrium while the second refers to the relationship to the serosa. One example is below
	2-5	Submucous and subserous, each with less than half the diameter in the endometrial and peritonealcavities, respectively.

Q2. What are atypical fibroids at locations outside the uterus?

Extrauterine may arise from anywhere where there is Mullerian tissue.

Broad ligament (True or Pseudo), Ovarian ligament, Uterosacral, Round ligament, Vulva, Vagina, Parasitic or Wandering.

Q3. What are parasitic myomas, diffuse leiomyomatosis peritonei and the difference between the two?

Parasitic myoma and diffuse leiomyomatosis peritonei are both rare types of uterine fibroids, but they have distinct characteristics and clinical implications.

Parasitic myoma: Parasitic myomas are a type of uterine fibroid that detach from the uterus and attach themselves to other structures within the abdominal cavity, such as the bowel, omentum, or bladder. This can happen either spontaneously or following surgical procedures like myomectomy or hysterectomy.

Characteristics of parasitic myoma:

- *Location:* These myomas are found outside the uterus, attached to other abdominal or pelvic organs.
- *Symptoms:* Symptoms can vary depending on the size and location of the myoma but may include pelvic pain, pressure, or gastrointestinal symptoms if they impinge on the bowel.
- *Diagnosis:* Diagnosis typically involves imaging studies such as ultrasound, CT scan, or MRI to identify the location and extent of the fibroids.
- *Treatment:* Surgical removal is usually the treatment of choice, especially if the myomas cause symptoms.

Diffuse leiomyomatosis peritonei: Diffuse leiomyomatosis peritonei is a condition characterized by the widespread presence of multiple smooth muscle tumors (leiomyomas) throughout the peritoneal cavity. This is a very rare condition and is considered a type of disseminated peritoneal leiomyomatosis (DPL).

Characteristics:

- *Location:* Multiple small leiomyomas are scattered throughout the peritoneal cavity.
- *Symptoms:* Symptoms may include abdominal distension, pain, and gastrointestinal disturbances. The extent of symptoms can vary based on the number and size of the tumors.
- *Diagnosis:* Imaging studies like ultrasound, CT scan, or MRI can be used for diagnosis, but a definitive diagnosis may require a biopsy to differentiate these tumors from other conditions such as metastatic cancer.
- *Treatment:* Treatment may involve hormonal therapy to reduce the size and number of fibroids, and surgical intervention might be necessary in some cases. Long-term follow-up is often required due to the potential for recurrence.

Comparison: Parasitic myoma vs. diffuse leiomyomatosis peritonei

	Parasitic myoma	***Diffuse leiomyomatosis peritonei***
Origin	Parasitic myomas originate as uterine fibroids that detach and reattach elsewhere	Diffuse leiomyomatosis peritonei involves multiple small leiomyomas scattered throughout the peritoneal cavity
Spread	Parasitic myomas are usually singular or few in number and attach to specific locations outside the uterus	Diffuse leiomyomatosis peritonei involves a more widespread distribution of tumors within the peritoneal cavity
Diagnosis	Imaging studies such as ultrasound, CT scan, or MRI to identify the location and extent of the fibroids	Imaging studies like ultrasound, CT scan, or MRI can be used for diagnosis, but a definitive diagnosis may require a biopsy to differentiate these tumors from other conditions such as metastatic cancer
Treatment	Surgical removal is usually the treatment of choice, especially if the myomas cause symptoms	Treatment may involve hormonal therapy to reduce the size and number of fibroids, and surgical intervention might be necessary in some cases
Follow-up	Follow-up, usually not required	Long-term follow-up is often required due to the potential for recurrence

Q4. What are the common symptoms of fibroids?

- Asymptomatic >25%
- *Menstrual abnormalities:*
    - AUB
    - HMB
    - Intermenstrual bleeding (metrorrhagia)
    - Polymenorrhea
- *Pain:*
    - Dysmenorrhea
    - Pelvic pain, pressure, discomfort
- Lump abdomen
- Urinary symptoms—retention, frequency, incontinence
- Bowl symptoms—constipation, irregular bowl habit
- Infertility
- Miscarriage
- Pregnancy complications

Q5. Which fibroids cause abnormal uterine bleeding and why?

Submucous fibroids (FIGO 0, 1, 2), especially those distorting the endometrial cavity, are the ones which most commonly cause abnormal uterine bleeding (AUB). Fibroids located in other areas of the uterus (FIGO 4-7) may also cause AUB.

There are various theories that have been postulated to explain the relationship between fibroids and AUB. They are as follows:

- Increased endometrial surface area and the presence of fragile and engorged vasculature in the peri-myoma environment. The increase in vascular flow observed along with these enlarged vessels can overcome platelet action.
- Research has shown that fibroids are associated with complex cellular and molecular changes which also has an impact on angiogenesis, alteration in vasoactive substrates and growth factors as well as alteration in coagulation.
- Transforming growth factor beta (TGF-β) is produced in excess in the endometrium in women with fibroids and is associated with reduced levels of plasminogen activator inhibitor-1 (PAI-1), thrombomodulin and antithrombin III.
- It is now thought that fibroids also impact the endometrial function, receptivity as a whole and not just the regions overlying the myoma(s). Some of these changes may have an impact on endometrial receptivity and implantation as well as on AUB.

Q6. What are the various degenerations one may encounter in fibroids?

Degeneration usually happens due to fibroids outgrowing their blood supply, rapid increase in the tumor size or hormonal changes.

The different types of degeneration are:

- *Hyaline*—most common, the leiomyomatous tissues are replaced with hyaline tissue. Hyaline tissue is characterized by the presence of homogeneous eosinophilic bands or plaques in the extracellular space, which represent the accumulation of proteinaceous tissue.
- *Cystic*— less common, occurs primarily in post-menopausal women and following hyaline degeneration. There is a reduction in blood supply which causes cells to degenerate and cystic spaces appear.
- *Myxomatous*—Cystic areas are seen with gelatinous material.
- *Red*—usually only during or after pregnancy. It results from hemorrhagic infarcts (dead tissues) of uterine fibroids.
- *Necrotic*—when parts of a fibroid or the entire fibroid become necrotic.
- *Fatty*—when fat deposition occurs in the fibroid tissue
- *Calcific*—calcareous deposits can be seen in the different

Q7. What are the common clinical features of degeneration in fibroids?

The common clinical features of degeneration are:

- Pelvic pain which can range from mild discomfort to severe cramping.
- *Vaginal bleeding or spotting*—the bleeding may range from spotting to heavy bleeding.
- *Pressure* sensation in the pelvic region.
- Pain during pregnancy is a hallmark symptom of fibroid degeneration
- Tenderness in the whole abdomen
- Fever with leukocytosis
- Decrease or shrinkage in the size of the tumor

While fibroid degeneration can cause distressing symptoms, it is essential to note that this process does not necessarily indicate a severe health concern.

BIBLIOGRAPHY

1. Berek JS. Berek & Novak's Gynaecology; 14th edition. Philadelphia: Lippincott Williams and Wilkins; 2007.
2. FIGO Leiomyoma Subclassification System, 2018.
3. Ghosh S, Naftalin J, Imrie R, et al. Natural History of Uterine Fibroids: a Radiological Perspective. Curr Obstetr Gynecol Rep. 2018;7:117-21.
4. Giuliani E, As-Sanie S, Marsh EE. Epidemiology and management of uterine fibroids. Int J Gynaecol Obstet. 2020;149(1):3-9.
5. Mukherji J. Basics of Gynaecology for Examinees, second edition. India: Academic Publisher; 2019. pp. 398-405.
6. Stewart EA, Cookson CL, Gandolfo RA, et al. Epidemiology of Uterine Fibroids: A Systematic Review. BJOG. 2017;124(10):1501-12.
7. Whitaker L Critchley HO. Abnormal Uterine Bleeding. Best Pract Res Clin Obstet Gynaecol. 2016;34:54-65.

CHAPTER 3

Myomas and Subfertility

Venugopal M, Basab Mukherjee

Q1. What is the prevalence of fibroids among the subfertile population?

Draft recommendations:

- *Fibroids are commonly seen in women across their reproductive age.*
- *Generally fibroids do not influence fertility but are diagnosed in 5–10% of women with infertility.*
- *Fibroids may be the sole cause of infertility in 2–3% of women.*

Uterine myomas (leiomyomata, fibroids) are the most common tumor of the reproductive tract, with a cumulative incidence of 70% in women across the reproductive age.

Fibroids are a common pathology and increasingly observed in women seeking medical treatment for infertility. The longer reproductive horizon because of improvements in medical care and current trend for women to postpone childbearing are making fibroid-related infertility increasingly common.

Q2. What is the impact of fibroids on reproductive outcome?

Draft recommendations:

- *Fibroids are associated with pregnancy loss - early and recurrent.*
- *Depending on their location, fibroids are associated with adverse obstetric outcomes.*

Fibroids distorting the uterine cavity typically affect implantation and cause higher miscarriage rates in the first and second trimester. Intramural fibroids have more effect on the functionality of the myometrium thus influencing preterm labor rates, placenta abnormalities, intrauterine growth restriction, increasing rates of caesarean section and postpartum hemorrhage. Besides these pain during pregnancy may be encountered in fibroids due to growth or degeneration changes.

Q3. What is the impact of fibroids on subfertility?

Draft recommendations:

- *The effect of subfertility depends on the fibroid size, position in the uterus and the alteration of the endometrial cavity*
- *Subserosal myomas have not shown to have a negative impact.*
- *For submucosal fibroids (types 0–2) surgical intervention is needed*

- *In intramural fibroids the degree of association with fertility depends on the degree of endometrium involvement and disruption of its contour.*

The relationship between fibroids and infertility has long been a topic of debate among gynecologists. The management of fibroids in women with otherwise unexplained subfertility lacks standard and evidence based guidelines. Subserosal fibroids do not appear to have an impact on fertility. If intramural fibroids have a less significant impact when the endometrium is not involved. The impact of the number of fibroids on subfertility has not been clearly elucidated. Studies have demonstrated conflicting reproductive outcomes related to the myoma size. While some studies support the notion that larger myomas more than 3 cm negatively impact reproduction, other studies suggest that myomas less than 5 cm in size do not.

Q4. What are the potential mechanisms by which fibroids cause subfertility?

Draft recommendations:

- *There are several hypotheses by which fibroids are believed to cause sub fertility ranging from genetic factors, mechanical compression, increased uterine contractions to inflammatory markers affecting implantation micro-environment adversely.*

Fibroids can cause sexual dysfunction as a result of dyspareunia, pelvic pain and heavy abnormal menstrual bleeding which could potentially interfering with sexual arousal and consequently the frequency of intercourse and subsequently a reduced probability of conception. Mechanical compression by fibroids situated around the interstitial part of the fallopian tubes or causing deformation of uterine cavity could disturb gamete transport. Fibroids may disturb the peristalsis of the junctional zone in the myometrium thus negatively influencing oocyte and sperm transport as well as implantation. In addition, fibroids could induce a detrimental environment for implantation by changing the vagino-uterine microbiome, disturbing the levels of inflammation and autophagy, inducing molecular changes in the endometrium, inducing aberrant angiogenesis and altering the endometrial blood supply.

Other mechanism of subfertility in fibroids includes genetic, cytokine factors and alteration of uterine contractions.

Q5. What are the indications of myomectomy in subfertility?

Draft recommendations:

- *Infertile women and those women undergoing Assisted Reproductive Technology (ART) procedures who have demonstrated submucous fibroids.*
- *Infertile women with symptomatic fibroids, such as heavy vaginal bleeding or pressure symptoms. No clear fertility benefit demonstrated.*

- *Couples presenting with multiple failed cycles of Assisted Reproductive Technology (ART) where the female partner has intramural fibroids.*

In women with infertility, an effort should be made to adequately evaluate and classify fibroids, particularly those impinging on the endometrial cavity, using transvaginal ultrasound, hysteroscopy, hysterosonography, or magnetic resonance imaging. (III-A) The utility of myomectomy thereafter needs to be individualized. In infertile women with symptoms, surgery is indicated for the symptoms but the positive impact on fertility is yet to be clearly ascertained. Indications for surgery should be clearly assessed esp. for intramural fibroids as scarring of the uterine wall can affect subsequent pregnancies. Removal of subserosal fibroids is not recommended. (III-D) Submucosal fibroids are managed hysteroscopically. The fibroid size should be <5 cm, although larger fibroids have been managed hysteroscopically, but repeat procedures are often necessary. (III-B) There is fair evidence to recommend against myomectomy in women with intramural fibroids not impinging on the endometrium and otherwise unexplained infertility, regardless of their size. (II-2D) If the patient has no other options, the benefits of myomectomy should be weighed against the risks, and management of intramural fibroids should be individualized. (III-C)

Q6. Does myomectomy improve subfertility?

Draft recommendations:

- *There is limited evidence to establish a clear benefit esp. for intramural fibroids.*
- *The location of the fibroid in an asymptomatic women clearly determine the benefit of myomectomy on reproductive outcomes.*
- *Myomectomy can cause adhesions both intra-abdominal and intra uterine which can adversely affect future pregnancies.*

In a Cochrane review, it was noted that limited evidence exists to determine the role of myomectomy for infertility in women with fibroids as only one trial compared myomectomy with no myomectomy. If the decision was taken to have a myomectomy, the current evidence does not indicate a superior method (lap'scopy or lap'tomy) to improve rates of live birth, preterm delivery, clinical pregnancy, miscarriage, or caesarean section.

In women with otherwise unexplained infertility, submucosal fibroids should be removed in order to improve conception and pregnancy rates.

Uterine incisions done posteriorly for posterior myomas have been found to be involved in more adhesions. They have potential to involve the ovaries and contribute to future fertility problems. There are guidelines from SOGC and CNGOF (France) to suggest an anterior uterine incision for a myoma approached through the abdominal route. For hysteroscopic resection the use of bipolar energy and anti-adhesion gel reduces adhesion risk and improves pregnancy rates.

Q7. How does myoma and myomectomy affect ART success rates?

Draft recommendations:

- *Submucosal and intramural fibroids that distort the endometrial cavity are associated with lower pregnancy, implantation and delivery rates in women undergoing IVF compared to infertile women without fibroids.*
- *FIGO type 3 fibroids not indenting the cavity may still have an deleterious effect if >3 cm in size.*

Intracavitary fibroids (submucosal and intramural distorting the cavity) negatively impact assisted reproductive outcomes. In a meta-analysis analyzing myomas negatively affect pregnancy rates, it was observed that submucosal lesions appear to strongly interfere with the chance of pregnancy OR (95% IC) of conception and delivery is 0.3 (0.1–0.7) and 0.3 (0.1–0.8).

A published review on the effect of fibroids on fertility with a meta-analysis reported that women with submucosal component had decreased clinical pregnancy and implantation rates compared with infertile control subjects.

A retrospective case-control study about the impact of FIGO type 3 fibroids on the outcome of IVF cycles reported that type 3 fibroids ≥30 mm might exert deleterious impact on implantation, clinical pregnancy and live birth rates of IVF cycles.

A meta-analysis about the impact of non-cavity distorting intramural fibroids on the efficacy of IVF included a total of 28 studies involving 9189 IVF cycles. They showed a significant reduction in LBR, CPR and implantation rate, and also have a significant increase in miscarriage rate compared with control group.

Q8. What is the role of non-surgical management of fibroids in patient with infertility?

Draft recommendations:

- *There is no role for medical management as a stans-alone treatment in the management of subfertile women with fibroids.*
- *Short term use of a GnRH analogue may be used for pre-operative correction of anemia or short term reduction in fibroid volume.*

Medication therapy is transient and is done essentially to control abnormal uterine bleeding. The current medical therapy is associated with suppression of ovulation, reduction of estrogen production and disruption of target action of estrogen or progesterone at the receptor level. It acts as a hindrance in the couple's ability to conceive. Hence there is no role for medical therapy as stand-alone treatment for fibroids in the infertile population.

Short term use of GnRH-a may be considered as a preoperative measure to reduce blood loss, decrease the size of the myoma and help to determine the route of surgery. Though the LNG IUS device controls bleeding it has limited effect on fibroid volume reduction. Selective Progesterone Receptor Modulators (SPRMs) like mifepristone and ulipristal have shown to reduce fibroid volume in women with symptoms but there are of no benefit in women with subfertility. Liver toxicity concerns remain for ulipristal which can be given in select populations.

Q9. Which are the novel methods of treatment of fibroids in infertile patients?

Draft recommendations:

- *It has been suggested that novel methods of treatment of fibroids should not be used outside the context of clinical trials in women desiring future pregnancies.*
- *There are lower pregnancy rates, higher miscarriage rates, and more adverse pregnancy outcomes following uterine artery embolization than after myomectomy. (II-3).*
- *Recent studies post MRgFUS reveal equivalent reproductive outcomes compared to laparoscopic myomectomy.*

Uterine Artery Embolization (UAE), MRgFUS, radio-frequency ablation (RFA), myolysis and uterine artery ligation should be used not be used outside the context of clinical trials in women desiring future pregnancies.

Uterine Artery Embolization (UAE) triggers ischemic necrosis in symptomatic fibroids and is highly effective for treating symptoms. A systematic review of pregnancy outcomes after fertility-sparing treatment of uterine fibroids reported high rates of successful pregnancies after myomectomy (75.6%) followed by ablation (70.5%). Post-UAE conceptions yielded the lowest live birth rates (60.6%) and highest miscarriage rates (27.4%). Studies also suggest that uterine artery embolization is associated with loss of ovarian reserve, especially in older patients. Women seeking future pregnancy should not generally be offered uterine artery embolization as a treatment option for uterine fibroids.

High-intensity focused ultrasound (HIFU) is a non-invasive ablative technique for myomas. Ultrasonic energy is directed at a point inside the fibroid and coagulation tissue necrosis is induced. HIFU is performed under the guidance of ultrasound or magnetic resonance (MRgFUS) Damage to surrounding tissue is minimal. It appears to be a safe and effective treatment in patients who wish to conceive with equivalent outcome in pregnancy rates compared to laparoscopic resection.

BIBLIOGRAPHY

1. Bai X, Lin Y, Chen Y, et al. The impact of FIGO type 3 fibroids on in-vitro fertilization outcomes: A nested retrospective case-control study. Eur J Obstet Gynecol Reprod Biol. 2020;247:176-80.

2. Baird DD, Dunson DB, Hill MC, et al. High cumulative incidence of uterine leiomyoma in black and white women: ultrasound evidence. Am J Obstet Gynecol. 2003;188:100-7.
3. Carranza-Mamane B, Havelock J, Hemmings R. The management of uterine fibroids in women with otherwise unexplained infertility. J Obstet Gynaecol Can. 2015;37(3):277-85.
4. Cook H, Ezzati M, Segars JH, et al. The impact of uterine leiomyomas on reproductive outcomes. Minerva Ginecol. 2010;62:225-36.
5. Cramer SF, Patel A. The frequency of uterine leiomyomas. Am J Clin Pathol. 1990;94:435-8.
6. Don EE, Mijatovic V, Huirne JAF. Infertility in patients with uterine fibroids: a debate about the hypothetical mechanisms. Hum Reprod. 2023;38(11):2045-54.
7. Donnez J, Dolmans MM. Hormone therapy for intramural myoma-related infertility from ulipristal acetate to GnRH antagonist: a review. Reprod Biomed Online. 2020;41(3):431-42.
8. Freytag D, Günther V, Maass N, et al. Uterine fibroids and infertility. Diagnostics. 2021;11:1455.
9. Giuliani E, As-Sanie S, Marsh EE. Epidemiology and management of uterine fibroids. Int J Gynaecol Obstet. 2020;149(1):3-9.
10. Jiang Z, Li Q, Li W, et al. A comparative analysis of pregnancy outcomes of patients with uterine fibroids after high intensity focused ultrasound ablation and laparoscopic myomectomy: A retrospective study. Int J Hyperth. 2021;38:79-84.
11. Khaund A, Lumsden MA. Impact of fibroids on reproductive function. Best Pract Res Clin Obstet Gynaecol. 2008;22:749-60.
12. Khaw SC, Anderson RA, Lui MW. Systematic review of pregnancy outcomes after fertility-preserving treatment of uterine fibroids. Reprod Biomed Online. 2020;40(3):429-44.
13. LaganàAS, Garzon S, Dababou S, et al. Prevalence of intrauterine adhesions after myomectomy: a prospective multicenter observational study. Gynecol Obstet Investig. 2022;87(1):62-9.
14. Luyckx M, Squifflet JL, Jadoul P, et al. First series of 18 pregnancies after ulipristal acetate treatment for uterine fibroids. Fertil Steril. 2014;102(5):1404-9.
15. Metwally M, Raybould G, Cheong YC, et al. Surgical treatment of fibroids for subfertility. Cochrane Database Syst Rev. 2020;1:CD003857.
16. Michos G, Dagklis T, Papanikolaou E, et al. Uterine Leiomyomas and Infertility: A Comparison of National and International Guidelines. Cureus. 2023;15(12): e50992.
17. Practice Committee of the American Society for Reproductive Medicine. Removal of myomas in asymptomatic patients to improve fertility and reduce miscarriage rate: a guideline. Fertil Steril. 2017; 108:416-25.
18. Pritts EA, Parker WH, Olive D. Fibroids and infertility: An updated systematic review of the evidence. Fertil Steril. 2009;91:1215-23.
19. Purohit P, Vigneswaran K. Fibroids and Infertility. Curr Obstet Gynecol Rep. 2016;5:81-8.
20. RANZCOG. (2018). Fibroids in infertility. Women's Health Committee. [online] Available from https://ranzcog.edu.au/wp-content/uploads/Fibroids-in-Infertility.pdf [Last accessed November, 2024].

21. Somigliana E, De Benedictis S, Vercellini P, et al. Fibroids not encroaching the endometrial cavity and IVF success rate: A prospective study. Hum Reprod. 2011;26(4):834-9.
22. Vilos GA, Allaire C, Laberge PY, et al. The management of uterine leiomyomas. SOGC Clinical Practice Guideline. J Obstet Gynaecol Can. 2015;37(2):157-78.
23. Wang X, Chen L, Wang H, et al. The Impact of Noncavity-Distorting Intramural Fibroids on the Efficacy of In Vitro Fertilization-Embryo Transfer: An Updated Meta-Analysis. BioMed Res Int. 2018;2018:1-13.
24. Zou M, Chen L, Wu C, et al. Pregnancy outcomes in patients with uterine fibroids treated with ultrasound-guided high-intensity focused ultrasound. BJOG. 2017;124:30-5.

CHAPTER 4

Imaging Modalities in Fibroids

Sunita Tandulwadkar, Rashmika Gandhi, Sejal Naik, Alok Sharma, Munjal Pandya

Q1. What are different diagnostic modalities to diagnose fibroid uterus, and which is best?

Draft recommendations:

- Transvaginal ultrasound (TVUS) is the first-line imaging modality for fibroid diagnosis due to its accessibility, cost-effectiveness, and diagnostic sensitivity.
- Magnetic resonance imaging (MRI) is the most accurate for complex cases requiring detailed mapping, particularly in pre-surgical evaluation or fertility-preserving surgeries.
- Hysteroscopy is considered the gold standard for diagnosing submucosal fibroids.
- Saline sonohysterography (SSG) and Hysterosalpingography (HSG) are useful adjuncts for evaluating endometrial cavity abnormalities.

Summary of evidence: Studies indicate that TVUS is the primary diagnostic tool for fibroids due to its ease of use and cost-efficiency. However, it may struggle with deep-seated or intramural fibroids. MRI offers superior accuracy for complex or multiple fibroids, atypical presentations, or fertility preservation cases. Hysteroscopy provides direct visualization, particularly for submucosal fibroids. SSG and HSG help evaluate uterine cavity distortions but are adjunctive tools rather than primary modalities.

Research gap:

- Limited comparative studies on the efficacy of SSG, HSG, and TVUS for fibroid diagnosis.
- Lack of clear guidelines for choosing diagnostic tools based on fibroid types or clinical scenarios.

Q2. What role does MRI play in the pre-surgical mapping of fibroids for fertility-preserving surgeries?

Draft recommendations:

- MRI is the imaging modality of choice for pre-surgical mapping in fertility-preserving surgeries due to its precise localization and detailed anatomical information.

- MRI is particularly recommended for assessing vascularity and differentiating fibroids from other pelvic masses.

Summary of evidence:

- MRI provides unparalleled sensitivity and specificity in detecting the size, location, and number of fibroids. It is indispensable in planning fertility-preserving surgeries, ensuring precise surgical resection while preserving normal uterine tissue. Studies highlight its utility in identifying vascularity and atypical features, facilitating optimal surgical outcomes.
- Three dimensional (3D) USG, while not as detailed as MRI, is a practical and cost-effective option that provides excellent visualization of the uterine cavity and myometrium. It can accurately assess fibroid size and location, particularly for submucosal and intramural fibroids. Unlike MRI, 3D USG is more accessible and can be performed in real-time during consultations. However, its effectiveness may be operator-dependent and less reliable in patients with obesity or large fibroids.

Comparison:

Feature	***MRI***	***3D USG***
Sensitivity	Higher for all fibroid types	Good, especially for cavity assessment
Vascularity Assessment	Excellent	Limited
Cost	Expensive	Cost-effective
Availability	Limited in some settings	Widely available
Operator Dependency	Low	High

MRI is the preferred choice for complex cases, while 3D USG serves as a suitable alternative when MRI is unavailable or impractical.

Research gap:

- Lack of cost-effectiveness studies comparing MRI to other modalities for pre-surgical mapping.
- Limited data on MRI's role in assessing fibroid recurrence risk post-surgery.

Q3. Can CT scan be used as an alternative to MRI?

Draft recommendations:

- CT scan is not recommended as a primary modality for fibroid diagnosis due to its inferior soft tissue contrast compared to MRI.
- It is reserved for cases where MRI is unavailable or when coexisting abdominal or pelvic conditions are being evaluated.

Summary of evidence: CT scans are limited in accurately characterizing fibroids. While they may detect large fibroids, their utility is compromised by lower soft tissue contrast. MRI remains superior for detailed evaluation and mapping, especially for fertility-preserving interventions.

Research gap:

- Need for research on the use of CT in combination with other modalities in settings without MRI access.
- Limited data on the diagnostic accuracy of CT in atypical fibroid presentations.

Q4. Can SSG or HSG be used for diagnosis of submucosal fibroids?

Draft recommendations:

- SSG and HSG are effective adjunctive tools for diagnosing submucosal fibroids, particularly in infertility evaluations.
- SSG is preferred over HSG due to its superior delineation of intrauterine abnormalities.

Summary of evidence: SSG uses saline infusion to enhance visualization of fibroids within the uterine cavity, offering better differentiation from other pathologies like polyps. HSG identifies uterine cavity distortions caused by fibroids but is less accurate than SSG for fibroid-specific diagnosis.

Research gap:

- Limited head-to-head comparisons of SSG and HSG in diagnosing submucosal fibroids.
- Need for studies on patient-reported outcomes when using SSG versus HSG.

Q5. What is the advantage of MRI over USG in diagnosis of intramural fibroids?

Draft recommendations:

- MRI is recommended over USG for diagnosing intramural fibroids due to its higher sensitivity and specificity.
- MRI is preferred in cases where detailed mapping or differentiation from other masses is necessary.

Summary of evidence: MRI excels in visualizing deep-seated intramural fibroids and provides detailed anatomical information, which USG cannot achieve due to limitations like acoustic shadowing or patient body habitus. MRI is particularly useful in planning surgical interventions or assessing atypical fibroid presentations.

Research gap:

- Need for cost-effectiveness studies comparing MRI and USG for intramural fibroids.

- Limited data on patient outcomes when using MRI for surgical planning.

Q6. Does the use of Doppler in TVS help in diagnosing characteristics of fibroids?

Draft recommendations:

- Doppler ultrasound is a valuable adjunct to TVUS for assessing vascularity and distinguishing fibroids from other pelvic pathologies.
- It is particularly useful in monitoring treatment response, such as uterine artery embolization.

Summary of evidence: Doppler ultrasound identifies vascularity patterns within fibroids, aiding in characterizing their growth and potential complications. Studies have shown its utility in distinguishing fibroids from adenomyosis and monitoring therapeutic interventions.

Research gap:

- Limited data on standardizing Doppler flow parameters for fibroid characterization.
- Need for studies on Doppler's role in predicting fibroid response to treatment.

Q7. Which is considered as a gold standard technique to diagnose the extent of submucosal fibroid in the uterine cavity?

Draft recommendations:

- Hysteroscopy is the gold standard for diagnosing and evaluating the extent of submucosal fibroids.
- It is also useful for determining the feasibility of surgical resection.

Summary of evidence: Hysteroscopy provides direct visualization of submucosal fibroids, enabling accurate diagnosis and treatment planning. It is particularly beneficial when imaging modalities like USG or MRI yield inconclusive results.

Research gap:

- Lack of studies comparing hysteroscopy with advanced imaging modalities for submucosal fibroid evaluation.
- Limited evidence on patient-reported outcomes following hysteroscopy.

Q8. Is there any use of AI in the detection of fibroids?

Draft recommendations:

- AI, particularly Deep Convolutional Neural Networks (DCNN), shows potential in enhancing fibroid detection and classification in imaging studies.

- AI applications can standardize diagnostics and reduce operator dependency.

Summary of evidence: Studies demonstrate that AI-driven tools improve diagnostic accuracy, especially in ultrasound imaging, by automating fibroid detection and reducing variability. Emerging evidence supports its integration into clinical practice for consistent and early diagnosis.

Research gap:
- Limited clinical trials on the effectiveness of AI in routine fibroid diagnostics.
- Need for cost-effectiveness and scalability studies for AI adoption in clinical settings.

BIBLIOGRAPHY

1. Dueholm M, Lundorf E, Hansen ES, et al. Accuracy of magnetic resonance imaging and transvaginal ultrasonography in the diagnosis, mapping, and measurement of uterine myomas. Am J Obstet Gynecol. 2002;186:409-15.
2. Murase E, Siegelman ES, Outwater EK, et al. Uterine Leiomyomas: Histopathologic Features, MR Imaging Findings, Differential Diagnosis and Treatment. Radiographics. 1999;19:1179-97.
3. Shahzad A, Mushtaq A, Sabeeh AQ, et al. Automated Uterine Fibroids Detection in Ultrasound Images Using Deep Convolutional Neural Networks. Healthcare. 2023;11(10):1493.
4. Shalev J, Meizner I, Bar-Hava I, et al. Predictive value of transvaginal sonography performed before routine diagnostic hysteroscopy for evaluation of infertility. Fertil Steril. 2000;73(2):412-7.
5. Wilde S, Scott-Barrett S. Radiological appearances of uterine fibroids. Indian J Radiol Imaging. 2009;19(3):222-31.

CHAPTER 5

Managing Asymptomatic Fibroids

Shehla Jamal, Annith Kumar VM

Q1. What are asymptomatic fibroids, and how common are they?

Draft recommendations: Asymptomatic fibroids, or myomas, are common in women, particularly as they approach menopause. They may be discovered incidentally during routine exams or imaging for unrelated issues. This document provides an overview of managing asymptomatic fibroids across different age groups and includes recommendations for follow-up and treatment.

Awareness and education:

- *Increase public awareness:* Inform women, particularly African-American women, about the high prevalence of fibroids (up to 80% by age 50) to encourage early detection and management.
- *Focus on age-related risk:* Educate women in their 30s and 40s about the increased risk of fibroids as they approach menopause.

Enhanced screening:

- *Routine screening for high-risk groups:* Consider regular ultrasound screenings for women at higher risk, even if asymptomatic, to detect fibroids early. Uterine fibroids are more common in women aged 30–40, particularly those of African American descent, with a family history of fibroids. Obesity, early menarche, high estrogen levels (due to factors like hormonal therapy or pregnancy history), and high blood pressure are additional risk factors. Diets high in red meat, vitamin D deficiency, and alcohol consumption may also increase risk. Fibroids are less common after menopause when estrogen levels drop.
- Having a family history of fibroids should be an important risk factor to recruit in screening.
- *Improve diagnostic accuracy and training:* Advocate for better imaging techniques to more accurately detect smaller fibroids, ensuring a true understanding of their prevalence.

Summary of evidence: Fibroids, also known as myomas, are prevalent in women, particularly as they near menopause. Studies show that African-American women have a 60% chance of developing fibroids by the age of 35, and this percentage increases to almost 80% by the age of 50. The prevalence of this condition among Caucasian women is 40% by the age of

35 and about 70% by the age of 50. These statistics indicate that the occurrence of fibroids tends to rise as individuals age until they reach menopause, at which point the development of new fibroids becomes uncommon.

An investigation utilizing meticulous serial sectioning of uteri from a sample of 100 women who underwent hysterectomy unveiled the presence of myomas in 77% of instances, with some as little as 2 mm. On average, premenopausal women had 7.6 myomas, whereas postmenopausal women had 4.2 myomas. Notably, myomas were equally common in women who had a hysterectomy for reasons unrelated to fibroids, but they were typically smaller in size and fewer in number.

The majority of women get fibroids during their reproductive years, regardless of whether they experience symptoms or not. It is frequently mentioned that 50% of fibroids do not show any symptoms; however, this estimation is probably too low. Several women with fibroids are often discovered coincidentally during tests for unrelated purposes and deny experiencing any symptoms connected to fibroids. Determining the actual prevalence of fibroids without symptoms is challenging.

The size, quantity, and placement of fibroids are important factors in determining whether they result in symptoms. Submucosal fibroids have a higher likelihood of causing excessive menstrual bleeding and bleeding between periods, although not all submucosal fibroids show symptoms. Pedunculated fibroids typically do not cause symptoms unless they experience torsion. Intramural fibroids commonly produce symptoms because they alter the shape of the uterine cavity. However, in certain cases, women may suffer symptoms such as excessive menstrual bleeding due to the fibroids growing larger, rather than causing distortion. The size at which fibroids induce symptoms varies, with some women having enormous fibroids but no symptoms, while others with smaller fibroids experience significant discomfort.

There are variations in how symptoms are perceived among individuals; certain women experiencing menorrhagia may view their menstrual periods as normal, while others may ascribe increasing urine frequency to the process of aging rather than fibroids. These ladies may be categorized as asymptomatic while experiencing symptoms.

Research funding for fibroids is disproportionately low compared to other non-malignant disorders, despite their great frequency. The reason for this is most likely because fibroids are non-cancerous, and many women do not experience any symptoms. Fibroids typically result in illness rather than death.

To summarize, although most fibroids do not show any symptoms, the often-cited statistics are probably lower than the actual numbers. The prevalence of fibroids varies between 20% to 77%. However, the actual frequency is likely greater because current imaging techniques have problems in detecting tiny fibroids.

Research gaps: Exact prevalence of asymptomatic fibroids is yet underestimated. Highlighting the frequency of occurrence along with secondary changes that may appear over the timeline of natural history of disease will guide for need for monitoring. To exactly evaluate as to how many asymptomatic variety will turn into symptomatic is also imperative.

Q2. How are asymptomatic fibroids typically discovered in clinical practice?

Draft recommendations:

- Detection during routine gynecological screening:
  - Incorporate regular pelvic examinations as part of routine gynecological care, especially for women aged 35–49, to identify potential abnormalities such as uterine fibroids. While pelvic exams alone may not confirm fibroids, they can prompt further diagnostic evaluation.
  - Encourage the use of ultrasonography, particularly transvaginal ultrasound, as a primary diagnostic tool for detecting fibroids, given its high sensitivity (95%) and specificity (85%). This is especially recommended for asymptomatic women during routine examinations.

Summary of evidence: Asymptomatic fibroids are often discovered by chance during regular medical examinations because they are benign and do not cause any symptoms but definitely raise concerns to the mind of the patients. Identifying these growths usually requires the use of various diagnostic methods.

During regular pelvic examinations, clinicians may identify abnormalities or notice an increase in the size of the uterus, which may require additional study. Pelvic examinations by themselves are not sufficient to definitively diagnose the existence of fibroids, but they can provide a first indication for further investigation.

Ultrasonography is a commonly used technique for detecting fibroids. There are two types of ultrasound procedures: transabdominal ultrasound and transvaginal ultrasound. Transvaginal ultrasonography is quite efficient in visualizing tiny fibroids. Research suggests that around 50–70% of women who have pelvic ultrasonography for reasons unrelated to fibroids are discovered to have fibroids. A study conducted by Baird et al., (2003) found that ultrasound screens detected fibroids in 51% of asymptomatic African-American women and 31% of asymptomatic Caucasian women aged 35–49. The sensitivity of ultrasound for detecting fibroids is 95%, meaning it accurately identifies 95% of cases. Additionally, it has a specificity of 85%, indicating that it correctly identifies 85% of cases where fibroids are not present (Stewart, 2001).

Furthermore, CT or MRI scans of the abdomen can detect asymptomatic fibroids, even when performed for other reasons.

Research gaps: Good quality and controlled data is unavailable to compare clinical evaluation with radiological diagnostic modalities. Longitudinal surveys, specially in Indian context are sparse. Majority of the fibroids are identified on symptom presentation. Exact incidence and identification of asymptomatic fibroids is still an enigma.

Q3. Can asymptomatic fibroids become symptomatic over time? If so, what are the factors that may contribute to this?

Yes and multiple factors contribute to the same.

Draft recommendations:

- *Clinical monitoring and symptom management:* Patients with fibroids should undergo regular clinical evaluations to monitor for growth and symptom development, especially during pregnancy, due to the risk of complications like red degeneration. Symptom management should address pelvic pain, urinary issues, and reproductive concerns.
- *Early detection of degenerative changes:* Special attention should be given to detecting early degenerative changes in fibroids, particularly red degeneration during pregnancy, to provide prompt interventions for pain control and minimize risks associated with hemorrhage and anemia.

Summary of evidence: It is observed that asymptomatic fibroids either grow and sometimes become large enough to produce symptoms, or undergo secondary changes and can manifest an array of symptomatology. The factors responsible for growth are hormones and their upregulation of receptors, vascular endothelial growth promotors, neoangiogenesis and endothelium promoters including IGF, platelet-derived factors, transforming growth factor alpha and basic fibroblast growth factor. All the above-cited growth factors are ligands of the well-known and established receptor tyrosine kinases (RTK) that activate two critical signaling cascades such as the Ras-Erk/MAP kinase and phosphatidylinositol-3 kinase (PI3K)-AKT-mTOR pathways. The mitogenic action of steroids in their target tissues is considered to be mediated by local production of growth factors acting through paracrine and/or autocrine mechanisms. The modulation of growth factor expression by steroids suggests growth factors represent the ultimate effectors of many steroid hormone actions. In addition to the genomic actions of steroid hormones on growth factor expression, non-genomic interactions of growth factors and hormone signaling pathways have also been demonstrated.

The symptoms produced by enlargement range from feeling of dragging in the pelvis, *anterior* symptoms related to bladder like frequency, retention of urine, recurrent UTI episodes owing to stasis of urine. *Lateral symptoms* include compression of ureters leading to hydro ureters and later on urosepsis. A few case reports of renal dysfunction owing to growing fibroids have also been reported. *Posterior symptoms* include bowel dysfunction mainly tenesmus and constipation. Deep dyspareunia has also been reported due to impacted Pouch of Douglas fibroids. *Caudal* symptoms arise when fibroid extends in cervicovaginal region and thus causing abnormal bleeding, subfertility.

Secondary changes, most notably, secondary degenerations occur in intramural fibroids. Various types have been recognized like hyaline, calcific, cystic fatty and sarcomatous. The one warranting special mention is Red Degeneration which occurs during pregnancy. Hyaline degeneration is most common and reported in 63% of cases. Cystic changes, the end result of hyaline degeneration, were observed by Rosai and Zaloudek and Hendrikson in 4.1% of cases. Fat cells, skeletal muscle, and cartilage have been identified in leiomyoma. It is not uncommon to find scattered adipocytes in an otherwise typical leiomyoma. Leiomyomas showing a striking amount of fat changes are called lipoleiomyomas. Red degeneration is a hemorrhagic infarction of the uterine leiomyoma, which is a well-known complication, especially during pregnancy. Red degeneration occurs in 8% of tumors complicating pregnancy, although the incidence rate can vary depending on the study.

Red degeneration results from hemorrhagic infarction within a leiomyoma, leading to severe pain and other symptoms. It usually manifests as acute abdominal pain, fever, and nausea. This condition can be managed conservatively with pain relief, as it often resolves on its own. Severe cases might require hospitalization or surgical intervention. The factors contributing to red degeneration include physical alterations like increasing size, decreasing central vascularity and resultant hypoxia.

Mavrelos et al. reported that the size of fibroids at the initial diagnosis is a significant independent predictor for subsequent fibroids growth ($p = 0.01$) with growth showing unilinear pattern.

Research gaps: The association between topography, size, number of fibroids and secondary changes is poorly understood. The data indicating larger fibroids undergoing secondary changes in more frequency is inconsistent. The type of change has been attributed to many factors such as Growth Hormone, VEGF, but the exact relationship is yet unexplored. On further researching, we can use these factors as bio markers for secondary changes, especially for Red degeneration and Sarcomatous change.

Q4. What should be the frequency and type of follow-up for fibroids managed expectantly?

Draft recommendations:

- No Treatment for Asymptomatic UFs: Emphasize that asymptomatic fibroids do not require treatment unless they show signs of significant growth or symptom development.
- Follow-up Strategy: Establish a follow-up schedule to monitor fibroid growth. Recommended intervals include 6 months for initial assessments, extending to 1 year if no growth is detected. For postmenopausal women, if fibroids remain stable for a year, they do not need further monitoring unless symptoms develop.

Summary of evidence: Asymptomatic fibroids do not generally necessitate treatment. Following up with periodic evaluations is recommended to monitor growth and detect potential changes. Guidelines suggest a follow-up schedule of 6 months, which may be extended to 1 year if no growth is noted. For postmenopausal women, fibroids that remain stable over a year generally do not require further monitoring unless symptoms arise.

The CNGOF guideline recommends annual imaging for large fibroids in women over 40. However, this recommendation is not strongly supported by evidence and highlights the need for further research. The frequency and type of follow-up should be tailored to individual cases, considering factors such as fibroid size, growth rate, and any associated symptoms.

Research gap: Frequency of monitoring in large and multiple fibroids is not precisely defined. Moreover in younger age group, females desiring future fertility and patients with concomitant pathologies like adenomyosis, fibroadenoma of breasts, the frequency is not mentioned.

Q5. How should asymptomatic fibroids be managed?

Draft recommendations:

- *Hysteroscopic resection for submucosal fibroids:* Hysteroscopic resection is recommended for women with asymptomatic submucosal fibroids that deform the uterine cavity, particularly for those seeking to improve fertility or if fibroids interfere with reproductive outcomes.
- *Management of asymptomatic intramural and subserosal fibroids:* Routine myomectomy for asymptomatic intramural or subserosal fibroids is generally not recommended unless symptoms develop or if there is a specific indication such as infertility.

Summary of evidence: Hysteroscopic myomectomy is a preferred treatment for symptomatic submucosal fibroids, offering a minimally invasive approach with high success rates. It is particularly beneficial for submucous myomas affecting the uterine cavity. In contrast, abdominal myomectomy may be less effective in certain cases and could result in leaving behind fibroids. In subfertile group, the approach is best tailored according to Lasmar classification. After resection of submucous myomas, both clinical pregnancy rates and live birth rates have been reported to improve. Pitts et al. investigated the impact of fibroids on fertility and impact of myomectomy. They concluded that submucosal myomas have a relative risk of 0.36 of achieving clinical pregnancy and a RR of 0.32 for the live birth when compared to the counterparts without fibroids.

When immediate fertility is a priority and one or more asymptomatic submucous myoma is detected having size >15 mm, hysteroscopic myomectomy should be offered. Cold loop resectoscope is preferred allowing healthy myometrium to be preserved.

The controversy of removing intramural myomas causing a positive impact on fertility stands as it is till date. For asymptomatic intramural and subserosal fibroids, routine myomectomy is not recommended unless symptoms arise or there is a clear indication. Management should be individualized based on the presence of symptoms and the impact on the patient's quality of life and reproductive health.

Research gap: The size and number of intramural fibroids that impact fertility is under researched. The efficacy of myomectomy in larger intramural asymptomatic fibroids and <15 mm submucosal asymptomatic, where immediate fertility is not desired is not clear and various authors have reported both favorable and unfavorable outcomes.

Q6. What are the potential risks associated with leaving them untreated?

Draft recommendations:

- *Psychological burden:* Provide clear communication about the benign nature of most fibroids and address patient concerns. Ensure that patients are informed about the low likelihood of malignancy and the typically manageable risks associated with untreated fibroids.
- *Malignancy risk:* While the risk of malignancy in fibroids is low, use ultrasound for initial diagnosis and consider advanced imaging if malignancy cannot be definitively ruled out. Regular monitoring is crucial to identify any changes.
- *Growth and compression:* Regularly monitor fibroid size and any symptoms that may develop. Consider intervention if significant growth or new symptoms occur.
- *Pregnancy and fertility:* Assess the impact of fibroids on pregnancy and fertility on an individual basis. Consider intervention for fibroids that cause complications during pregnancy or impact fertility.

Summary of evidence: Untreated asymptomatic fibroids may lead to psychological distress, although they are generally benign. There is a low but real risk of malignancy, which can be managed with appropriate imaging and monitoring. Growth and compression issues may occur, leading to potential symptoms and complications. Regular monitoring is important to manage these risks effectively.

During pregnancy, fibroids may cause complications, and their impact on fertility should be assessed individually. In cases where fibroids cause significant issues or complications, appropriate intervention should be considered.

Cho et al. retrospectively reviewed 31 women who developed leiomyosarcoma. They observed BMI <20, largest fibroid diameter >8 cm as independent predictive risk factors for leiomyosarcoma with sensitivity of 41–63.3% for BMI and 82.4% for largest lesion. Seki and associates explored the use of LDH and its isozyme, LDH 3 as the best negative predictors for Leiomyosarcomas.

Research gap: Majority data for secondary changes NAD degeneration comes from symptoms appearing in asymptomatic fibroids. Clinical studies have indicated that leiomyosarcoma can appear independent of fibroid as well. Prospective data on utilization of biomarkers is lacking, thus to enhance the current knowledge more prospective recruitment of asymptomatic subjects is required.

BIBLIOGRAPHY

1. Baird DD, Dunson DB, Hill MC, et al. High cumulative incidence of uterine leiomyoma in black and white women: ultrasound evidence. Am J Obstet Gynecol. 2003;188:100-7.
2. Cho HY, Kim K, Kim YB, et al. Differential diagnosis between uterine sarcoma and leiomyoma using preoperative clinical characteristics. J Obstet Gynaecol Res. 2016;42(3):313-8.
3. Mas A, Tarazona M, Dasí Carrasco J, et al. Updated approaches for management of uterine fibroids. Int J Womens Health. 2017;9:607-17.
4. Mazzon I, Favilli A, Grasso M, et al. Predicting success of single-step hysteroscopic myomectomy: a single-center large cohort study of single myomas. Int J Surg. 2015;22:10-4.
5. Saridogan E. Surgical treatment of fibroids in heavy menstrual bleeding. Womens Health (Lond). 2016;12(1):53–62.
6. Seki K, Hoshitara T. Leiomyosarcoma of the uterus: ultrasonography and serum lactate dehydrogenase level. Gynecol Obstet Invest. 1992;33(2):114-8.
7. Vilos GA, Allaire C, Laberge PY, et al. The management of uterine leiomyomas. SOGC Clinical Practice Guideline. J Obstet Gynaecol Can. 2015;37(2):157-78.
8. Vitale SG, Riemma G, Ciebiera M, et al. Hysteroscopic treatment of submucosal fibroids in perimenopausal women: when, why, and how? Climacteric. 2020;23(4):355-9.

CHAPTER 6

Myomas and Pregnancy

Anahita Chauhan, Anupama Dave

Q1. How common are myomas associated with pregnancy and in which demographic profiles?

- Prevalence of myomas in pregnancy varies between 1.6 and 10.7%, depending upon which trimester of pregnancy it was reported, the size and the demographic characteristics of the population.
- The prevalence varies with race and increases with maternal age.
- Reduction of prevalence is seen with increasing parity and prolonged breastfeeding.
- Fibroids are three times more common in black women compared to other populations; similar incidence is seen in Hispanic, Asian and white women.

Q2. How do existing myomas affect pregnancy?

Draft recommendations:

- The majority of women do not have any pregnancy complications related to their fibroids.
- A slightly increased risk of early pregnancy loss, preterm labor and birth, fetal malpresentation, and placental abruption has been reported. However, studies have not consistently reported an increased risk of adverse outcomes.
- High-quality data on the relationship between fibroids and pregnancy outcomes is minimal.

Summary of evidence: Myomas are associated with higher rates of miscarriage in the first trimester. One study found higher miscarriage rates in those with fibroids (14%) than those without (8%). Rarely, fibroids are associated with fetal anomalies, possibly caused by compression effects from large submucosal fibroids. Structural anomalies including limb reduction defects, dolichocephaly and torticollis have been reported.

Q3. Role of preconceptional myomectomy?

Draft recommendations:

- The decision to do a myomectomy in the preconception period must be made on a case-by-case basis and depend on several factors, including the age of the patient, past reproductive history, the severity of symptoms, and the size, number and location of the fibroids.

- Myomectomy should be performed in cases where there is a submucosal myoma or cavity distorting intramural myomas.
- Myomas of 5 cm or more even non cavity distorting should be removed especially if elderly lady, low ovarian reserve and no other obvious factors identified causing infertility.

For details, please refer to section 'Surgical Management of Fibroids'.

Q4. Role of myomectomy in the antenatal period?

Draft recommendations:

- *Antepartum abdominal myomectomy*—indications include intractable pain and fever, or a pedunculated fibroid with torsion. Ideally, it should be done in the second trimester.
- *Antepartum transvaginal myomectomy*—rarely may be done may be done for clinically significant bleeding, unmanageable pain, urinary retention, and (rarely) infection during pregnancy due to a prolapsed fibroid.

Summary of evidence: There is consensus to avoid myomectomy during pregnancy, especially if an intramyometrial incision is required unless the procedure cannot be safely delayed, which is extremely rare. The reason is that the inability to control bleeding during intramyometrial myomectomy is a real possibility and may necessitate a hysterectomy. These rare scenarios may include an acute abdomen, obstruction, and suspicion of malignancy

Q5. What effect does pregnancy have on fibroids, the risks associated and their management?

- Fibroid may remain the same or increase in size during pregnancy.
- It may be more likely in the first trimester than the third trimester.
- Fibroids located close to the lower segment may migrate upwards with advancing pregnancy.
- Rapidly growing fibroids may be associated with red degeneration and pain, and pedunculated fibroids may undergo torsion.

Summary of evidence: Despite a high prevalence of fibroids, scarce information is available on the influence of maternal characteristics on fibroid growth during pregnancy and there are no meta-analysis. Mitro et al., 2022 conducted a secondary analysis of a prospective cohort study of 2,774 women with singleton pregnancies who underwent 6 antenatal ultrasounds (NICHD fetal growth study-singleton). Overall, 9.6% (266/2,774) of women had a visualized fibroid at any time during pregnancy, including 9% (67/745) of non-Hispanic white women, 14% (106/770) of non-Hispanic black women, 6% (47/794) of Hispanic women (NHW), and 10% (46/465) of Asian or Pacific Islander women. The mean total fibroid volume decreased by 1.0% (95% confidence interval [CI], –1.9%, –0.2%) per week, with a variation in starting total volume. On average, the total volume increased by 2.0% (95% CI, –0.3%, 4.5%) per week among women with small volume; decreased by 0.5% (95% CI, –2.0%, 1.0%) per week among women with medium volume; and decreased by 2.2% (95% CI, –3.4%, –1.0%) per week among women with large volume at first visualization. The volume change also varied by race or ethnicity, parity, age, and miscarriage history studies demonstrated changes in fibroids during pregnancy, often with growth during the first trimester and variable growth or regression in the later trimesters.

Q6. How do you routinely monitor patients with myomas during pregnancy?

Draft recommendations:

- Regular ultrasonographic surveillance is required for the identification of rapidly enlarging fibroids.
- Sometimes sonography may be needed to relocate the myoma as a cause for fetal malpresentation in the latter stages of pregnancy.

Research gap: There are no studies mentioning this aspect specifically but pregnancy being monitored as a high risk pregnancy.

Q7. What is the role of Cesarean Myomectomy?

Draft recommendations:

- The decision to perform a myomectomy during a cesarean section should ideally be made preoperatively. Informed consent of the patient and her relatives should be taken.
- Myomectomy is necessary at cesarean birth when the myoma is at the uterine incision site where otherwise, it would be difficult to close the uterine wound. In other cases, it should be individualized.
- Cesarean myomectomy can be considered electively or opportunistically by a surgeon who has the appropriate expertise, and there is the availability of blood products, in appropriately selected cases (e.g., symptomatic pedunculated fibroids).
- In cases of multiple and large-sized myomas CM should be preferred over CS alone, especially by experienced surgeons with appropriate hemostatic techniques and tertiary care centers.
- Cesarean myomectomy may be safe and feasible in selected patients with myomas, regardless of size and location, except if they are located at the cornual end or close to large vessels, and in the absence of uterine atony during surgery. [Huang Y et al., 2022]

Summary of evidence: In a meta-analysis of mostly retrospective studies of patients with myomas who had concomitant myomectomy at Cesarean, had greater drops in hemoglobin, an approximately 40% increase in the use of blood transfusion, and longer hospital stay.

Another systematic review and meta-analysis of observational studies showed no increased rate of major bleeding or need for transfusion. According to them, cesarean myomectomy may be considered in cases of isolated myomas, although randomized trials are needed. Intramural myomas, myomas ≥7 cm in size, and multiple myomas are associated with more intraoperative hemorrhage and prolonged operation duration. With appropriate hemostatic techniques and when performed by experienced surgeons CM may be considered. It is especially useful in low resource settings so as to avoid an interval myomectomy.

Q8. Choosing the route of delivery in pregnant women with fibroids and a history of previous myomectomies

Draft recommendations:

- Patients without prior myometrial surgery can have a successful vaginal birth and thus should be offered a trial of labor. Cesarean birth is reserved for standard obstetric indications.
- Planned cesarean birth may be considered because of concerns that fetal descent will be obstructed by a fibroid, those with large cervical fibroids or with lower uterine segment fibroids that distort the uterine cavity and are located between the fetal vertex and cervix in the third trimester.
- Patients with prior myomectomy—timing and route of delivery must be individualized based on the degree and location of the prior uterine surgery. If during myomectomy full thickness of myometrium was incised Cesarean Birth before the onset of labor is advised.
- If trial of labor is given: Continuous intrapartum fetal monitoring, early access to obstetric anesthesia, and the ability to perform an emergency cesarean birth in emergency
- Prior hysteroscopic removal of a submucosal fibroid may increase the risk of abnormal placentation, especially the placenta accreta spectrum.

Summary of evidence: Available data suggest that a trial of labor after myomectomy could perhaps be as safe (or as risky) as a trial of labor after cesarean delivery, as the incidence of uterine rupture in labor with a trial of labor after myomectomy is 0.47% and the incidence of uterine rupture for the trial of labor after cesarean delivery in labor is about 0.5–1%. These data suggest that a trial of labor after myomectomy might be considered a feasible and possible safe option for pregnant women with prior myomectomy and that these women may be treated similarly to those with prior CD. This has been reported in a systematic review of studies with at least five cases of pregnancy after myomectomy.

Q9. What are the technical issues in cases with myoma during pregnancy during a cesarean birth?

Draft recommendations:

- During Cesarean section precautions should be taken especially in patients with large, retroplacental or anterior lower uterine segment fibroids who are at increased risk of intrapartum or postpartum hemorrhage.
- Preoperative placement of two large bore IVs, use of a cell saver, and ready availability of blood products should be considered on a case-by-case basis.
- A vertical (midline) skin incision may be necessary in some cases to obtain adequate exposure.
- Ultrasound imaging can be used (either antepartum or intrapartum) to map out the optimal location for the hysterotomy incision at the time of cesarean in patients with large uterine fibroids. Intraoperatively, a sterile probe cover is placed on the ultrasound transducer and sterile gel is applied to the uterine serosa; the best incision site can then be mapped sonographically.
- Every effort should be made to avoid transecting a fibroid during hysterotomy as the incision may be impossible to close without first removing the fibroid. Even with a myomectomy, it may be impossible to close the incision in such cases, necessitating a hysterectomy.

Q10. What complications are expected in the postpartum period and their management? What contraception can be advised?

- Complications of fibroids in the postpartum period are extremely rare
- Pyomyoma is a life-threatening complication resulting from infarction and infection of fibroids.
- There is no difference in regression based on age, parity, body mass index, level of education, income, smoking, size and location of fibroids, mode of delivery, postpartum infection, breastfeeding, or time for the return of menstruation.

Concerns with postnatal/Interval contraception:

- As per WHO medical eligibility criteria, all methods of contraception are safe and can be used in the postpartum or interval period.
- In case the patient is breastfeeding, COC should be used with caution for the first 6 months (category 2).
- In case the patient has a submucous fibroid or a fibroid distorting the endometrial cavity, copper IUD and LNG IUS are contraindicated (category 4).

Q11. What are the concerns of pregnancy after a myomectomy?

- The risk of a uterine rupture in pregnancy following a myomectomy, regardless of the technique, is less than 1% of ongoing pregnancies.
- Women with Caesarean myomectomy in a previous pregnancy are at higher risk of placenta previa, abnormal lie and talipes in the next pregnancy.
- The risks, and the inherent danger of bleeding with placenta previa, should be taken into consideration when evaluating the benefit of Cesarean myomectomy to avoid a later interval myomectomy.

Summary of evidence: The outcome of pregnancies following a previous caesarean myomectomy has been studied. The spontaneous pregnancy rate is as high as 79.3% following a caesarean myomectomy, in marked contrast to interval myomectomy, which has quoted rates of between 38.6 and 55. A study of 29 women showed a mean interpregnancy interval of 31.2 months following caesarean myomectomy; 20.7% required fertility treatment in the form of clomiphene, division of intrauterine adhesions and hydrogenation for distal tubal occlusion.

Limitations of available evidence research gaps: Several factors make it difficult to assess the impact of fibroids on pregnancy outcomes and to identify important specific fibroid characteristics. For example, the interpretation of available evidence is limited by the heterogeneity of the study populations, which differ in the method of ascertainment (e.g., prospective versus retrospective study design), gestational age at diagnosis, and fibroid characteristics (number, size, location [fundus, lower uterine segment], type [submucosal, intramural, subserosal; pedunculated or sessile]). Small numbers of adverse events, ascertainment bias in selecting study participants, and inadequate adjustment of confounders also play a role. In addition, small fibroids (<4 to 5 cm) may not be detected consistently because they can be difficult to distinguish from physiologically thickened myometrium. Lastly, the mechanisms whereby fibroids may cause adverse obstetric outcomes are not clearly understood.

BIBLIOGRAPHY

1. Coutinho LM, Assis WA, Spagnuolo-Souza A and Reis FM. Uterine Fibroids and Pregnancy: How Do They Affect Each Other? Reproductive Sciences. 2022:29; p. 2145.
2. Gambacorti-Passerini Z, Gimovsky AC, Locatelli A. Trial of labour after myomectomy and uterine rupture: a systematic review. Acta Obstetricia et Gynecologica Scandinavica. 2016;95:724.

3. Ghosh S, Naftalin J, Imrie R, et al. Natural History of Uterine Fibroids: a Radiological Perspective. Curr Obstetr Gynecol Rep. 2018;7:117-21.
4. Goyal M, Dawood AS, Elbohoty SB, et al. Cesarean myomectomy in the last ten years; A true shift from contraindication to indication: A systematic review and meta-analysis. Eur J Obstetr Gynecol Reprod Biol. 2021;256:145-57.
5. Hammoud AO, Asaad R, Berman J, et al. Volume change of uterine myomas during pregnancy: do myomas grow? J Minim Invas Gynecol. 2006;13:386-90.
6. Huang Y, Ming X, Li Z. Feasibility and safety of performing cesarean myomectomy: a systematic review and meta-analysis. J Matern Fetal Neonat Med. 2022;35(13):2619-27.
7. Mitro S, Peddada S, Chen ZG, et al. Natural history of fibroids in pregnancy: NICHD Fetal Growth Studies—Singletons cohort. Fertil Steril. 2022;118:656-65.
8. Neiger R, Sonek JD, Croom CS, et al. Pregnancy-related changes in the size of uterine leiomyomas. J Reprod Med. 2006;51:671-4.
9. Pergialiotis V, Sinanidis I, Louloudis IE, et al. Perioperative Complications of Cesarean Delivery Myomectomy: A Meta-analysis. Obstetr Gynecol. 2017;130(6):1295-303.
10. Sampat K, Alleemudder DI. Fibroids in pregnancy: management and outcomes. Obstetr Gynaecol. 2018;20:187-95.
11. Spyropoulou K, Kosmas I, Tsakiridis I, et al. Myomectomy during pregnancy: A systematic review. Eur J Obstetr Gynecol Reprod Biol. 2020;254:15.
12. Stewart EA, Cookson CL, Gandolfo RA, et al. Epidemiology of Uterine Fibroids: A Systematic Review. BJOG. 2017;124(10):1501-12.

7

CHAPTER

Medical Management of Fibroids

Shobha N Gudi, Monika Anant

INTRODUCTION

In contemporary gynecological practice there are multiple modalities of treatment for fibroid uterus. The factors determining the modality (embolization, medication, or surgery) depends upon patient preferences depending on tolerance to side effects), invasive nature of treatment (surgery UAE), recovery time, need for prolonged treatment (more than 6 months), risk of the treatment vs recurrence, availability and cost.

Q1. What are the indications for medical management?

Draft recommendations:

- Symptomatic patients with heavy menstrual bleeding not desiring fertility
- Fibroids which are not located in sub-mucosal region (FIGO type 0, 1, and 2)
- Symptomatic patients with bulk or pain symptoms with or without bleeding (preoperative as a size reduction therapy or transitional therapy for patients in late perimenopause)

Summary of evidence: There were no RCT/meta-analysis for the indications of medical therapy found.

Clinical practice points are women with not desiring fertility. The symptoms of heavy menstrual bleeding, bulk or pain of the sub-mucosal site require medical treatment.

Q2. Which cases are suitable for medical management?

Most of the medical therapies available for uterine fibroids are not suitable for women desiring fertility as many preclude conception, long-term use can cause adverse effects, and result in rapid symptom rebound when discontinued.

- All women who are symptomatic due to fibroids which are not exclusively sub-mucosal are good candidates.
- In women who do not desire immediate fertility all options of medical management are directed towards reducing Heavy menstrual bleeding/ bulk and pain symptoms.
- Patients who also have bulk, pain or pressure symptoms are directed to medical treatment options that can reduce fibroid size as well.
- Finally, some patients are unwilling for surgery and are given medical therapy.

Summary of evidence: There are no data to compare the options of available medicines, so choice is with consideration of efficacy, safety, tolerability, ease of use, and cost.

Q3. What structured counseling must be undertaken before start of medical therapy?

Draft recommendations:

- Counseling of patients with leiomyomata improves patient satisfaction and knowledge.
- Counseling must be undertaken only after complete evaluation of the fibroids is done, first with history on symptoms of HMB, pain, pressure and fertility issues, information on numbers, size, location with adequate imaging, (3D USG if possible). Associated co morbidities like obesity, diabetes, menopause or perimenopause.
- Suggested counseling points for patients with fibroids:
  (a) What are fibroids?
  (b) What causes fibroids?
  (c) Where can fibroids grow? (Figure can be added)
  (d) What are symptoms of fibroids?
  (e) How the presence of fibroids is confirmed?
  (f) What happens in pregnancy with fibroids?
  (g) Can fibroids turn into cancer?
  (h) What are the treatment options for fibroids?
  (i) What new treatments are available for uterine fibroids?

The information for therapy must be provided:

- Hormone therapy is used to give relief from heavy menstrual bleeding and period pain. There can be some reduction in size but not complete cure. The effect is only during the use of hormones.
- Side effects and adverse effects of medical management must be discussed. Patient must be informed that hot flashes and impact on BMD happens with specific therapies (e.g., GnRH analogs) but will be counteracted by the additional add back hormones, lifestyle modification, anemia correction, calcium and vitamin D supplements and regular follow-up.
- Medical therapy is an option for women just before menopause - or for women for whom surgery is contraindicated.

Summary of evidence: Medical management has transient impact so the fibroids may grow again once it is stopped. Hormonal therapy before surgery will correct anemia and reduce size and vascularity of fibroids so surgery is easier.

Q4. Any pretreatment evaluation required.

Draft recommendations:

- Associated morbidities, e.g., anemia must be treated for better efficacy of the medical management.

- Information on volume and location of tumors (fibroid mapping) aids in treatment planning and follow-up for response.
- Identify concomitant disease e.g., uterine sarcoma/endometrial hyperplasia/cancer.
- Significant hydronephrosis due to ureteral obstruction by a fibroid uterus must be alleviated and needs surgical removal or bulk reducing medication.
- In general, women considered for hormone therapy, and in particular when Ulipristal acetate is considered must have evaluation with detailed history for past or current liver disease and a thorough assessment of liver function tests.

Summary of evidence: Important to check whether location consistent with bulk-related symptoms of pelvic pain or pressure, urinary symptoms, bowel symptoms. If initial evaluation suggests malignancy, MRI imaging, Doppler USG three-dimensional (3D)/four-dimensional (4D) studies and histopathology is mandatory to exclude malignancy.

Q5. What are the treatment options for managing fibroids medically?

Draft recommendations:

- High dose Progestins are used to treat HMB due to fibroid for a short or intermediate period (grade C).
- Progestogen treatment of HMB due to fibroids, levonorgestrel intrauterine system LNG-IUS is validated for use, administered by the endouterine route (grade B).
- Tranexamic acid is effective for HMB due to fibroids (grade B).
- Pain associated with fibroids to be treated with NSAIDs (grade B).
- Use GnRH analogs for short period (3 months) in preoperative management, to reduce bleeding and correct anemia. (LE1).
- GnRH antagonists also relieve menorrhagia/dysmenorrhea (LE2).
- Mifepristone reduces fibroid size and improves the symptoms. (LE1).
- Ulipristal acetate is used as intermittent treatment of HMB due to uterine fibroids in premenopausal women who are not suitable for surgery or uterine artery embolization. Daily 5 mg dose of UPA can be given for up to four courses of treatment only.
- The use of danazol is not recommended, due to side effects and short duration of efficacy (grade C).
- In women needing contraception but with cavity distortion which precludes the use of LNG-IUS, low dose combined oral contraceptives are effective for symptom relief and are prescribed with MEC criteria for short periods of six months.

Summary of evidence: Progestin-only contraceptives Cochrane review concluded that oral progestins did not reduce fibroid size or fibroid-related symptoms. High-dose oral progestins do not appear to be as effective for treatment for fibroid-related HMB as the LNG IUD.

LNG IUS is suitable for fibroids less than 3 cm in diameter, not causing distortion of the uterine cavity. Combined oral contraceptives are not contraindicated for fibroids. A recent meta-analysis suggests they control HMB in uterine fibroids with no effect of increasing fibroid volume. A systematic review reported that tranexamic acid is more effective than oral progestins. NSAIDs reduce pain/dysmenorrhea associated with fibroid, though there are no controlled trials for the same.

Mifepristone reduced heavy menstrual bleeding and improved quality of life reduce fibroid volume as seen in 3 RCTs. **Ulipristal acetate** offers similar advantages (reduced fibroid volume bleeding and improved anemia). It is indicated for some premenopausal women. [If surgery for fibroids is not feasible. **GnRH analogs** reduces uterine and fibroid volume. GnRHa also increase preoperative hemoglobin levels, although hot flushes are bothersome. During hysterectomy, blood loss, operation time and complication rates were also reduced. There is no reliable evidence available from RCT for benefits of the use of **danazol** or **aromatase inhibitors** or **SERMs**, e.g., **Raloxifene** for uterine fibroids.

Despite evidence supporting use of the progesterone receptor modulators (PRM) ulipristal acetate and mifepristone for fibroid-related bleeding, neither is currently available in most countries for fibroid treatment; and in settings where these drugs are available, use is restricted given potential for hepatic toxicity. SERM raloxifene use as hormonal add-back with GnRH analog treatment for fibroids appeared to reduce bone loss but did not improve quality of life.

Q6. What is the ideal follow-up care planned for such cases?

Draft recommendations:

- A symptom diary or menstrual calendar with record of bleeding, pain and pressure symptoms to be maintained by patient. Any new symptom as weight loss, fatigue, increasing pressure symptoms must be reported.
- Periodic imaging (USG)to determine size of fibroids, degeneration, vascularity, concomitant disease emergence like adenomyosis and endometrial hyperplasia.

Q7. Which medical treatment works better and how long should the treatment be continued?

Draft recommendations:

- Effective medical treatments for women with AUB-L include the levonorgestrel intrauterine system, (I) gonadotropin-releasing hormone analogs, (I) selective progesterone receptor modulators, (I) oral contraceptives, (II-2) progestins, (II-2).

- Effective medical treatments for women with bulk symptoms associated with fibroids include selective progesterone receptor modulators and gonadotropin-releasing hormone analogs. (I)
- Can continue using NSAIDs and/or tranexamic acid for as long as they are found to be beneficial.

Discussion: Effective medical therapy reduces the need for surgery and may be cost-effective. However, fibroid recurrence rate of 50% once therapy is matter of concern.

NSAIDs, Tranexamic acid and COCs as long as benefited by symptomatic relief.

LNG-IUS to be used till its date of effectivity (5 years).

GnRH agonists can be used for 2–3 months.

GnRH antagonists: Relugolix combination therapy was approved up to *24 months.*

SPRMs: Mifepristone: 3–6 months, Ulipristal Acetate treatment if used pre-operatively or premenopausal is limited to three months of continuous use.

Summary of evidence: Relugolix combination therapy—Relugolix-estradiol-norethindrone was approved by the US FDA in May 2021 for the treatment of fibroid-related HMB for up to *24 months.*

Q8. What are the common side effects of medical therapy?

Draft recommendations: Prolonged treatments with drugs like GnRH analogs, Ulipristal is to be carefully monitored for side effects.

- Tranexamic acid increases the rate venous thromboembolism, infarct-type necrosis and thrombosis of leiomyoma
- NSAIDS, *COCs usual side effects amenable to treatment.*
- *LNG-IUS:* Minimal side effects of irregular bleeding which settles within 3–6 months of insertion.
- SPRMs UPA: cases of serious liver toxicity, liver transplantation, and fatalities have been reported.
- There is increased *abnormal endometrial histology (PAEC) but is benign and reversible after discontinuation.*
- *GnRH agonist* significant hypoestrogenic side effects (hot flashes, sleep disturbances, vaginal dryness, depression), including bone loss.
- *GnRH antagonists:*
  Elagolix combination therapy: Night sweats and reductions in bone mineral density.
- *Relugolix combination therapy:* Hypersensitivity reactions (e.g., anaphylaxis, urticaria, angioedema) have been described.

Summary of evidence: To minimize the risk of the rare but serious liver injury with UPA: It is contraindicated in women with known liver problems;

LFT before, during, and after stopping treatment; should not be used more than one treatment course unless surgery is not feasible.

Elagolix combination therapy (mean reduction of 4.8 percent at the end of 12 months of treatment, with improvement to reduction of 2 percent one year following completion of treatment).

Q9. What is the role of gonadotropin-releasing hormone (GnRH) agonists and antagonists in treating fibroids?

GnRH analogs—GnRH agonists and antagonists constitute effective second tier medical treatments: to reduce fibroid-associated HMB.

Agonists also reduce fibroid volume but have potential adverse effects.

GnRH antagonists—once the first-tier medical treatment fails, oral GnRH antagonist combinations (with low dose estrogen and progestin) must be started. They act centrally and are associated with hypoestrogenic side effects, but are available as oral formulations with low-dose steroidal hormonal add-back to limit hypoestrogenic side effects,

- **Elagolix combination therapy** with estradiol and norethindrone is effective for treatment of fibroid-related HMB. Two capsules: One contains elagolix 300 mg plus estradiol 1 mg plus norethindrone 0.5 mg for the morning, and the other elagolix 300 mg at night for 6 to 12 months. The side effects are few but effect on volume reduction is poor due to add back therapy. This therapy does not reliably suppress ovulation, it should not be considered a contraceptive. When estrogen is contraindicated, e.g., hypertension or history of DVT: elagolix alone, without add-back therapy, improves fibroid-related HMB.
- **Relugolix combination therapy**—each tablet (single daily dose) contains relugolix + estradiol + norethindrone acetate (40 mg + 1 mg + 0.5 mg). The advantages of once daily dosing and greater reduction of pain and bulk symptoms, improved anemia and emotional wellbeing, no significant bone loss makes it suitable. Some Hypersensitivity reaction has been reported.
- **Linzagolix**—an oral GnRH antagonist: 100 mg (partial suppression) or 200 mg [full suppression hypothalamic-pituitary-ovarian (HPO) axis] of once daily tablet and has the option of being administered with or without add-back therapy.

GnRH agonists:

- These are used as transitional therapy for peri-menopausal HMB due to fibroids to relieve symptoms till they attain menopause thereby avoiding surgery.
- As preoperative therapy (for three months) for induction of amenorrhea to improve anemia when response to Iron therapy is inadequate and

for volume reduction to facilitate a less invasive route for hysterectomy, (vaginal rather than abdominal hysterectomy).

- IM Depot injection one to three months. causes significant hypo-estrogenic side effects, including bone loss and must be used with add-back therapies: Steroidal or nonsteroidal to limit side effects and allow long-term use,

Steroidal add back:

- Nonsteroidal add back therapy, herbal remedies, SSRI, SNRI.
- In addition: Weight bearing exercise, calcium, and vitamin D supplementation must be followed.
- For patients with main symptoms of bulk or pain, UAE or GnRH analogs is considered balancing availability, procedure risk, longer recovery with UAE as against hypoestrogenic symptoms with long-term use of GnRH analogs.

Summary of evidence: All GnRH antagonists seem to be equally effective with safety data for up to two years but not yet available for use in India. The side effects with **Elagolix plus add back therapy**: hot flushes, night sweats, headache, nausea, elevated liver transaminase levels in less than 10% of cases and needed discontinuation rarely only for LFT derangement. A small change of Bone mineral density (1.5%) regained after one year by 50%.

Approved by the US FDA May 2020 for 24 months of use.

Elagolix alone compared with placebo resulted in relief of HMB in 89% of patients and volume reduction by >50% after 12 months of therapy with mean reduction 4.8% BMD and gain back of 2% per year.

In two phase III trials evaluating **linzagolix therapy** for the fibroid-related HMB, significantly more patients treated with linzagolix (with or without 1 mg estradiol and 0.5 mg norethisterone acetate add-back therapy) showed relief. (MBL ≤80 mL and ≥50 %volume reduction from baseline at 24 weeks) compared with placebo.

In two phase III trials comparing 24 weeks of **relugolix combination therapy** (40 mg of relugolix, 1 mg of estradiol, and 0.5 mg of norethindrone acetate), and placebo, more patients in the treatment arms achieved MBL <80 mL, 50 % reduction in MBL compared with placebo (80 % versus 19 %). Rare events of Hypersensitivity reactions (e.g., anaphylaxis, urticaria, angioedema) have been described.

For patients with fibroids and anemia: Preoperative GnRH agonist treatment plus iron is an established option.

GnRH agonists decrease fibroid volume, increase hemoglobin, and improve perioperative outcomes in patients undergoing hysterectomy and myomectomy. Significant hypoestrogenic side effects, including bone loss makes add back therapy mandatory.

Q10. Do combination therapies have a role? What are the safety issues?

Draft recommendations:

- Tranexamic acid for period management and cyclical COC can be used together.
- Once-daily relugolix combination therapy (40 mg of relugolix, 1 mg of estradiol, and 0.5 mg of norethindrone acetate) resulted in a significant reduction in menstrual bleeding.

Summary of evidence: Concerns about an increased risk of venous thromboembolism (VTE) when combined hormonal contraception and tranexamic acid are combined, are not supported by long term clinical experience, the benefits of therapy for most women will outweigh potential risks.

Women with increased risks for VTE beyond the risk conferred by combined hormonal contraception (immobility, obesity, coagulopathy, etc.) should avoid this combination therapy.

Elagolix with hormonal add-back therapy is effective in reducing heavy menstrual bleeding associated with uterine fibroids independent of age, body mass index, race, ethnicity, baseline menstrual blood loss, fibroid location, and uterine and primary fibroid volume.

Q11. What is the rationale behind using SPRM's in the medical management of fibroids?

Facts: SPRMs have action at 3 levels

1. *Fibroids:* Inhibits cell proliferation and increases apoptosis
2. *Endometrium:* Benign and reversible changes in endometrium and leading to stoppage of uterine bleeding (PRM associated endometrial changes PAEC)
3. *Pituitary:* Maintains mid follicular phase of estradiol—anovulation—amenorrhea

Q12. What are indications of cessation of therapy in favor of operative intervention?

Draft recommendations:

From clinical experience:

- For patients who do not desire future fertility and have persistent fibroid-related symptoms despite a fair trial of medical therapy of 6 months.
- Growth of fibroids in spite of medical treatment
- Patients who desire surgical treatment
- Emergence of other gynec disease like endometrial hyperplasia with atypia.

BIBLIOGRAPHY

1. Al-Hendy A, Lukes AS, Poindexter AN 3rd, et al. Treatment of Uterine Fibroid Symptoms with Relugolix Combination Therapy. N Engl J Med. 2021;384:630.
2. Dailymed. (2023). MYFEMBREE-relugolix, estradiol hemihydrate, and norethindrone acetate tablet, film coated. US FDA approved product information. [online] Available from: www.dailymed.nlm.nih.gov [Last accessed November, 2023].
3. Donnez J, Taylor HS, Stewart EA, et al. Linzagolix with and without hormonal add-back therapy for symptomatic uterine fibroids: 2 randomised, phase 3 trials. Lancet. 2022;400:896.
4. Eder S, Baker J, Gersten J, et al. Efficacy and safety of oral tranexamic acid in women with HMB and fibroids. Womens Health (Lond). 2013;9(4):397-403.
5. Ke LQ, Yang K, Li J, et al. Danazol for uterine fibroids. Cochrane Database Syst Rev. 2009;2009(3):CD007692.
6. Lethaby A, Puscasiu L, Vollenhoven B. Preoperative medical therapy before surgery for uterine fibroids. Cochrane Database Syst Rev. 2017;11(11):CD000547.
7. Liu JP, Yang H, Xia Y, et al. Herbal preparations for uterine fibroids. Cochrane Database Syst Rev. 2013;2013(4):CD005292.
8. Management of Symptomatic Uterine Leiomyomas: ACOG Practice Bulletin, Number 228. Obstet Gynecol. 2021;137(6):e100-e15.
9. Murat Naki M, Tekcan C, Ozcan N, et al. Levonorgestrel-releasing intrauterine device insertion ameliorates leiomyoma-dependent menorrhagia among women of reproductive age without a significant regression in the uterine and leiomyoma volumes. Fertil Steril. 2010;94(1):371-4.
10. Murji A, Whitaker L, Chow TL, et al. Selective progesterone receptor modulators (SPRMs) for uterine fibroids. Cochrane Database Syst Rev. 2017;4(4):CD010770.
11. NICE. (2020). Heavy menstrual bleeding: Assessment and management. [online] Avialable from https://www.nice.org.uk/guidance/ng88/resources/heavy-menstrual-bleeding-assessment-and-management-pdf-1837701412549 [Last accessed November, 2024].
12. Osuga Y, Enya K, Kudou K, et al. Relugolix, a novel oral GnRH antagonist, in the treatment of pain with uterine fibroids: a randomized, phase 3 study in Japanese women. Fertil Steril. 2019;112:922.
13. Qin J, Yang T, Kong F, et al. Oral contraceptive use and uterine leiomyoma risk: a meta-analysis based on cohort and case-control studies. Arch Gynecol Obstet. 2013;288(1):139-48.
14. Sangkomkamhang US, Lumbiganon P, Laopaiboon M, et al. Progestogens or progestogen-releasing intrauterine systems for uterine fibroids. Cochrane Database Syst Rev. 2013 ;(2):CD008994.
15. Tosun AK, Tosun I, Suer N. Comparison of LNG device with oral progestins for (HMB) with leiomyoma Pak J Med Sci. 2014;30:834.
16. Tristan M, Orozco LJ, Steed A, et al. Mifepristone for uterine fibroids. Cochrane Database Syst Rev. 2012;2012(8):CD007687.

CHAPTER 8

Surgical Management of Fibroids

8.1 OPEN MYOMECTOMY

Poushali Sanyal

Q1. What are the indications where open myomectomy is the preferred option over other routes?

Draft recommendations: Open myomectomy may be preferred over other routes in the following situations:

- Limited endoscopic skill set of the surgeon—where the surgeon is not trained or confident in performing a laparoscopic myomectomy.
- Extremely large or multiple or difficult to approach or remove laparoscopically.
- Sometimes with extreme adhesions or scarring of the patient's abdomen from previous surgeries or abdominal pathologies.
- Patient preference, when the patient, after knowing the risks and benefits of each route sometimes opts for an open surgery.
- Cardiopulmonary complications that are contraindications to general anesthesia, which is a prerequisite for laparoscopic myomectomy.

Evidence: Often, multiple prior abdominal surgeries cause significant abdominal adhesions and limit the scope of laparoscopic myomectomy. In such cases, open myomectomy is the preferred option. Sometimes, after knowing the risks with each route, the patient prefers an open myomectomy. Surgeons who are not that experienced in performing a myomectomy though the laparoscopic route should perform an open myomectomy keeping in mind the safety of the patient.

Q2. What are the surgical principles to be followed during an open myomectomy?

Draft recommendations: The surgical principles include:

- Proper patient selection based on the size, number, and location of the fibroids
- Careful preoperative planning by a thorough review imaging to locate and map the fibroids, and plan the surgical approach so that there is minimal blood loss during surgery.
- Obtain a written informed consent from the patient which has documented benefits, risks, alternatives and expected outcome of the procedure.

- Utilize various measures to control blood loss, such as Trendelenburg position during surgery, preoperative GnRh analog or Mifepristone, and 400 microgram misoprostol prior to surgery.
- Give proper antibiotic prophylaxis at the time of induction of anesthesia to contain postoperative infection.
- Administer appropriate anesthesia which minimizes blood loss, like spinal anesthesia.
- Avoid multiple uterine incisions and remove the fibroids via a single uterine incision, preferably avoiding the posterior uterine wall, to avoid post operative scarring and adhesions.
- Handle the tissues gently, use less diathermy, and secure proper hemostasis with barbed sutures or 1-0 V loc sutures for closing uterine incisions. Use of oxidized regenerates cellulose is not mandatory, but may be used as an antiadhesion agent during myomectomy.
- Proper closure of uterine incisions to promote proper wound healing and tension free stitches during uterine closure prevent pocket formation between sutures and prevent dehiscence of the uterine wound and post operative hemorrhage.

Proper patient selection for open myomectomy is the key to a successful surgery. Before starting the procedure, a preoperative MRI to locate and map the size of the fibroids helps to plan the surgical approach, cause minimal blood loss during surgery, and preserve the uterus. A written informed consent from the patient prior to starting the procedure explaining clearly the risks, benefits, outcome and alternatives is mandatory. Preoperative antibiotic prophylaxis during induction of anesthesia needs to be given to control post operative infection. Appropriate anesthesia to control blood loss like spinal anesthesia, Trendelenburg position prior to surgery, and 400 mcg of vaginal misoprostol prior to surgery are all measures to reduce intraoperative blood loss. Gentle tissue handling and proper hemostasis during surgery reduces the risk of postoperative adhesions. Barbed sutures are used to close the uterine incisions for better hemostasis and proper wound healing as these sutures provide tension free stitches and prevent formation of pockets in between the suture points.

Q3. What are the advantages of open myomectomy?

Draft recommendations: The advantages of open myomectomy over other routes are as follows:

- Preserving the uterus helps the woman conceive in future
- Complete removal of the fibroids frees the woman from symptoms like menorrhagia and dysmenorrhea
- The surgeon has a good ability to access and remove multiple fibroids at inaccessible locations like large cervical or broad ligament fibroids.

- There is a lower risk of complications as the surgeon has a better view of the surgical site, and for surgeons who are not that confident in endoscopy, there is a reduced risk of injury to surrounding organs like the bowel, bladder, and ureter.
- It requires a shorter operating time than laparoscopic or robotic myomectomy and involves less costs.
- In women with medical co morbidities where general anesthesia is difficult to use, and shorter operating time is mandatory, open myomectomy is the method of choice.
- There is a potential for improved outcomes like lower rate of fibroid recurrence compared to laparoscopic or hysteroscopic myomectomy.

Open myomectomy allows for the removal of fibroids while preserving the uterus, making it a suitable option for women who wish to maintain their fertility. It provides the surgeon with direct access to the fibroids, allowing for thorough removal and reducing the risk of recurrence. This procedure effectively addresses multiple fibroids of varying sizes and locations within the uterus. The open approach provides the surgeon with a clear view of the surgical site, reducing the risk of injury to surrounding organs such as the bladder or bowel. It is associated with a lower risk of complications compared to laparoscopic or robotic myomectomy. The open technique is recommended usually for women with larger fibroids located in challenging areas of the uterus that may be difficult to access using minimally invasive techniques. It has a shorter operating time compared to other procedures, which is helpful for women with medical co morbidities, and it may result in improved outcomes, such as reduced rates of fibroid recurrence.

Q4. What are the intraoperative complications during open myomectomy?

Draft recommendations: Some potential intraoperative complications during open myomectomy include:

- Excessive bleeding from uterine wall which may even lead to hysterectomy
- Injury to surrounding structures like bladder, ureter, intestines, and blood vessels
- Abdominal or surgical site infection
- Formation of pelvic adhesions
- Uterine rupture
- Anesthetic complications such as allergy, or lung atelectasis
- Post operative complications such as pain, deep vein thrombosis or delayed wound healing

Open myomectomy can sometimes lead to blood loss, particularly if a large fibroid needs to be removed or if there are multiple fibroids present. During the removal of fibroids, there is a risk of unintentional injury to adjacent organs. The formation of pelvic adhesions as a result of the surgery can lead to pain or other complications in the future like subacute intestinal obstruction. In rare cases, the uterus may rupture during the procedure, particularly if there is significant scarring or weakness in the uterine wall. It is important for the surgical team to carefully monitor the patient during the procedure and take steps to minimize the risk of these complications.

Q5. What are the post operative problems faced after open myomectomy?

Draft recommendations: In addition to infection, pelvic and incision site pain, bleeding, pelvic adhesions and damage to adjacent organs like the bladder, bowel and ureters, there is a possibility of recurrence of fibroids after surgery, and infertility in future due to extensive pelvic adhesions in the post operative period.

Studies confirm that women undergoing open myomectomy require a higher dose of post operative analgesics to control pain, have higher pain scores, and have a higher risk of post operative pelvic adhesions, particularly if the uterine incision is given on the posterior uterine wall or there are multiple uterine incisions. If the fibroids are not removed completely, there is a risk of recurrence of fibroids in future. Moreover, if the uterine cavity is opened during the procedure, especially in case of large or multiple fibroids, uterine synechiae, and future pelvic adhesions may render the women infertile in future.

Q6. When can a woman become pregnant after open myomectomy?

Draft recommendations: The woman can try for conception 3 to 6 months after an open myomectomy, depending on the individual's body healing process. It is important to follow the doctor's instructions and wait until the body has healed sufficiently to reduce the risk of complications during pregnancy.

A woman can become pregnant after open myomectomy once she has fully recovered from the surgery and her doctor gives her the go-ahead to try to conceive. It typically takes 3 to 6 months.

Q7. What is the risk of uterine rupture in a pregnancy after open myomectomy?

Draft recommendations: The risk of uterine rupture after an open myomectomy is estimated to be around 0.5 to 3 %. However, it is important to note that the actual risk can vary from individual to individual.

Studies have shown that the risk of uterine rupture in a pregnancy after an open myomectomy is generally low (0.5 to 3%), but it is higher than the baseline risk of uterine rupture in women without a history of prior uterine surgery (1%).

8.2 SURGICAL ASPECTS OF HYSTEROSCOPIC MYOMECTOMY

S Krishnakumar, Shrutika O Makde

Q1. Does the classification of the submucous myomas help in operative hysteroscopic myomectomy?

Draft recommendations:

- Before hysteroscopic myomectomy it is mandatory to classify the fibroids along with the size and volume which allows us to indicate the degree of difficulty and complexity of the surgery. A good transvaginal sonographic mapping is enough in majority of the cases and MRI is indicated if the number of fibroids increases beyond 5 or if another fibroid is suspected to be close to the submucous fibroid which probably could be close to the serosa.
- Type 0 and type 1 submucous myomas (ESGE) are more likely to be completely removed in a 1-step approach; conversely, large type 1 and type 2 submucous myomas could require a multistage procedure.
- In complex cases it is better to use the STEP W classification and should follow the following scoring guideline and approach:
  - 0 to 4 I low complexity hysteroscopic myomectomy.
  - 5 to 6 II complex hysteroscopic myomectomy, consider preparing with GnRH analog and/or 2-step surgery.
  - 7 to 9 III recommend an alternative non-hysteroscopic technique.

Summary of evidence: Among USG, Hysterosonography and MRI, Ultrasonographic mapping has good accuracy, easy access, low cost and helps to evaluate the free myometrial mantle which allows us to indicate the degree of difficulty and complexity of hysteroscopic myomectomy and the comparison of results.

Transvaginal ultrasound should be the first line to evaluate the number, size, and location of submucous myomas, with subsequent in-office hysteroscopy to allow, when feasible, a see-and-treat approach. The Lasmar-STEP-W classification provides a standardized approach to submucosal hysteroscopic myomectomy to minimize the risk

Lasmar submucous myoma classification—STEP-W classification (2005).

	Size	***Penetration***	***Base***	***Topography***	***Lateral wall***
0	≤2 cm	0	≤1/3	Lower	+1
1	>2 to 5 cm	≤50%	>1/3 to 2/3	Middle	
2	>5 cm	>50%	>2/3	Upper	
Score		+	+	+	
Score	*Group*	*Suggested treatment*			
0 to 4	I	Low complexity hysteroscopic myomectomy			
5 to 6	II	Complex hysteroscopic myomectomy, consider preparing with GnRH analog and/or 2-step surgery			
7 to 9	III	Recommend an alternative non-hysteroscopic technique			

Small <3 cm type 0 and 1 submucosal myoma can be removed in the office setting using hysteroscopic scissors or tissue removal systems with higher successful completion rates in a 1-step approach. Type 2 submucous myomas may require incision of pseudocapsule during office hysteroscopy protruding the fibroid in the uterine cavity increasing the likelihood of complete rection in subsequent sitting as a multistage procedure.

Q2. What are the techniques for hysteroscopic myomectomy and is the conventional enucleation of myoma always possible by hysteroscopy?

Draft recommendations:

- The different techniques used for hysteroscopic myomectomy depends on the size, location, penetration of myomas into the myometrium as given by Lasmar classification as well as experience of surgeon in the same.
- The present recommendation to perform hysteroscopic myomectomy is by the enucleation technique identifying the pseudocapsule wherever possible for better healing and reducing the chances of IU adhesions.
- The techniques of hysteroscopic myomectomy are Traditional Slicing Technique, Morcellation and Retrieval by Tissue retrieval system and Enucleation from the pseudocapsule—conventional myomectomy.

Summary of evidence and discussion:

Traditional slicing (Fragmentation): This is done using resectoscope-Monopolar (Outdated) or Bipolar with progressive cutting of the submucosal portion of the myoma and planned loop movements always in the fundus-cervical direction, with the angulation of the resectoscope axis to define the degree of resection depth **(Fig. 1)**. The speed of movement of the loop determines the action of more cutting or more coagulation; the faster moving

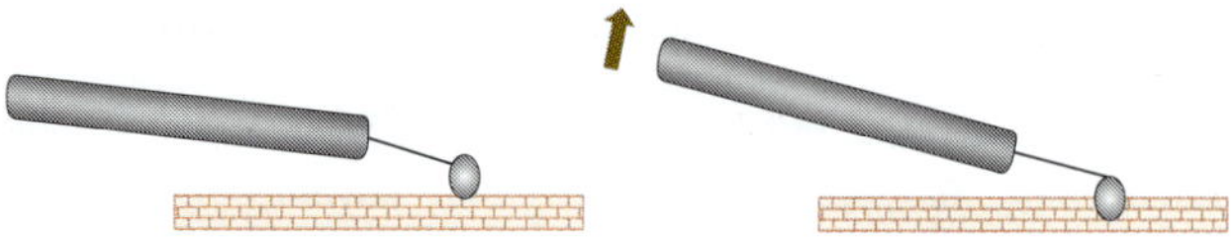

Fig. 1: Slicing technique demonstrating the effect of angulation of resectoscope on tissue depth.

loop cuts more and coagulates less, while the slower one coagulates more than it cuts.

The fragmented tissues remain within the cavity until retrieved leading to crowding of tissues.

Morcellation and retrieval: This technique performs fragmentation and suction of the submucosal fibroid, mainly used for type 0 and 1 myoma. This technique uses only mechanics as the energy source and eliminates the need for removal of resected fibroid chips from the cavity, hence shown to be faster and practicality of use looks simpler with a short learning time. Though their use is challenging in dense and calcified fibroids, deep type 2 fibroids and high cost of equipment.

Enucleation technique: Enucleation technique is known and performed by all gynecologists, in laparotomy or laparoscopy. When dissection is done along the pseudocapsule, the chance of preserving the uterus is greater, with decreased bleeding and myometrial damage. This involves incision of the endometrium around the submucosal myoma to reach the pseudocapsule (Lasmar) or to reach this plane by slicing the myoma close to the myometrium (Mazzon). On reaching the pseudocapsule, some fibrous beams are cut and the myoma is progressively freed from the myometrium using scissors and grasper or Collins "Cold" loop. As the myometrial vessels are not cut, the risk of intravasation, bleeding and myometrial damage is low. This is the recommended surgical approach in submucous myomas with an intramural component (FIGO type 1 and 2) to keep the pseudocapsule of the myoma intact, maintain the anatomic and functional integrity of the myometrium.

Gubini's technique involves the use of the mini resectoscope to incise the endometrium around myoma followed by changeover to the sturdier cold loop and gradually separating the fibroid from the surrounding fibers by pushing and sliding.

Some of the HTRS systems allow the use of 4 mm scissors through their operative bridge to make incisions making the myomectomy much easier and faster.

Among the different available hysteroscopic techniques, cold loop resectoscopic myomectomy is the favored approach as it preserves maximum healthy myometrium than other hysteroscopic myomectomy techniques, such as dissection, vaporization, or morcellation by hysteroscopic tissue removal systems. Finally, the use of a 16 F miniresectoscope, when available, should be considered.

Q3. What are the disadvantages of the slicing technique in hysteroscopic myomectomy?

Draft recommendations:

- *Time-consuming:* The slicing technique can be laborious, especially for large fibroids, leading to longer procedure times.
- *Risk of fluid overload:* The use of large volumes of irrigation fluid during the procedure can increase the risk of fluid overload and associated complications, such as hyponatremia.
- *Lack of tissue for pathological examination:* The slicing technique often results in fragmented tissue, making it difficult to obtain a complete specimen for histological evaluation.
- Overcrowding of myoma fragments in the uterine cavity, necessitating to interrupt the procedure with emptying of the cavity to retrieve myoma bits leading to frequent interruption of surgery.
- *Potential for uterine perforation:* The use of the cutting loop can increase the risk of uterine perforation, especially in cases with thin-walled fibroids or previous uterine surgery.

Summary of evidence and discussion: Slicing technique involves progressive removal of the myoma in fragments from the surface to the base. The greater thermal use increases the chances of greater removal or damage to the endometrium and myometrium with higher risk of intravasation of hysteroscopic distension media as the superficial vessels open up. During the procedure, overcrowding of myoma fragments in the uterine cavity occurs, causing frequent interruption in the procedure for emptying of the cavity to retrieve myoma bits. There is greater bleeding with greater possibility of intravasation causing incomplete myomectomy, risk of perforation and longer operative time.

The advantages include the ability to surgically treat larger nodules, and perform volumetric reduction along with achieving hemostasis at the same time. Due to these potential drawbacks, it is recommended that the slicing technique be considered in conjunction with other hysteroscopic myomectomy techniques, such as laser ablation or morcellation, to select the most appropriate approach for individual patients.

Q4. Is the hysteroscopic tissue retrieval system the best way to perform a hysteroscopic myomectomy?

Draft recommendations: Depending on the size, location, and number of fibroids, the HTRS involves removing the fibroid intact, preserving the uterine cavity and fragmenting the fibroid into smaller pieces before removal.

Summary of evidence and discussion: The HTRS is better due to practicality of use, short learning time, and non-use of energy (only mechanics). It has good performance in the treatment of intracavitary lesions and it alleviates the need for removal of fibroid "chips" from the cavity.

The disadvantages of the HTRS include high cost of the disposable element, as well as the difficulty resecting fundal fibroids and deep type 2 fibroids. Also, with HTRS, resection of dense and calcified fibroids can be very challenging requiring change to resectoscope in such instances. It has no chances of achieving hemostasis in presence of bleeding.

Q5. In cases where the myoma is separated from the attachment what are the ways of retrieving the same?

Draft recommendations:

1. Visual inspection and retrieval of a smaller myoma can be done by hysteroscopic grasper
2. Resection of myoma in small pieces and retrieval by HTRS is also an effective way.

Summary of evidence and discussion: Smaller myomas of less than 10 mm may be removed with strong graspers. When the myoma is larger it can be retrieved either by HTRS systems or resected with the help of resectoscope. The myoma can be left behind inside the cavity to shrink and atrophy, and subsequently be expelled after a couple of weeks. A follow-up sonography is to be done to confirm the same.

Q6. In cases where the myomectomy is incomplete how soon the second sitting be performed?

Draft recommendations:

- *Immediate follow-up:* To assess the extent of the incomplete removal and discuss the need for a second procedure.
- *Expectant management:* For small residual fibroids and mild symptoms, expectant management may be done considering the patient's condition and symptoms over time.
- *Second procedure:* The need for second procedure depends on the patient's symptoms and the size of the residual myoma:
- *Within a few months:* For larger or strategically located residual fibroids that are causing significant symptoms.
- *After conservative management:* If the residual fibroids are small and the patient's symptoms are manageable, conservative management is to be considered for 3 months to allow for potential spontaneous regression and stabilization.

Summary of evidence and discussion: 15.5–40% patients remained symptom-free after incomplete removal of submucous myoma. In patients with symptoms including heavy bleeding, the lack of symptoms is the endpoint, whereas in patients seeking pregnancy the endpoint is a normal uterine cavity free of residual myoma fragments. According to study conducted by Dueholm et al. if the patient is symptom free 3 months of conservative approach should be taken before the reoperation during which the residual tissue would disappear. Periodic ultrasound monitoring of these patients should be done. When there is a relative urgency of creating a normal uterine cavity, though the length of time to follow before repeating the procedure is not clear, follow-up ultrasound should be obtained in at least 3 months.

Q7. In a patient for future fertility treatment is there a need of relook hysteroscopy post hysteroscopies myomectomy?

Draft recommendations: In patients with infertility, outpatient second-look hysteroscopy is indicated 45 to 60 days after surgery to review the uterine cavity and lyse the adhesions seen during the procedure, with scissors or with the simple passage of the hysteroscope.

Summary of evidence and discussion: In a retrospective study conducted by Mazzon et al. the risk of IUA formation and need for relook hysteroscopy is low when using combination of monopolar energy and cold knife resection for myomectomy. The incidence of adhesion formation being 30%, a relook hysteroscopy to review the uterine cavity can be done after 45-60 days after the myomectomy.

Q8. Is outpatient hysteroscopic myomectomy safe and always feasible?

Draft recommendations: The safety and feasibility depend on:
- *Size and location of fibroids:* Smaller submucosal fibroids are more suitable for outpatient procedures. Large or deeply embedded fibroids may require a longer operating time or hospitalization.
- *Patient's overall health:* Women with underlying health conditions or a history of bleeding disorders may require additional precautions or hospitalization.
- *Procedure complexity:* If the procedure involves multiple fibroid removals or adhesion lysis, it may be more challenging to perform on an outpatient basis.

Summary of evidence and discussion: Hysteroscopic myomectomy in an outpatient setting is a safe procedure with lower cost compared to surgery in a hospital environment. However, patient discomfort and tolerability, unfavorable factors including fundal fibroid, size more than 2 cm, penetration in the myometrium may limit this procedure.

Safe to excise by office hysteroscope are the submucous myomas <15 mm located entirely inside the uterine cavity (type 0, as per FIGO).

The most preferred technique in outpatient myomectomy is enucleation technique with dissecting the endometrium around the fibroid with scissors, most commonly and occasionally with Collins knife using miniresectoscopy. This is followed by dissection using graspers or cold loop electrodes to separate it from the pseudocapsule. If the size of the fibroid is larger than the diameter of the internal os the fibroid can be retrieved with the HTRS system or left behind to be expelled spontaneously at a later stage.

Type 2 fibroids can be prepared first in office by incising the endometrium around the fibroid and partially enucleating it and can be completed during a second hysteroscopy with the resectoscope in 1 to 2 months, with intracavitary myoma (the OPPIuM Technique).

Q9. Is there a role of preoperative medical therapy

Draft recommendations: For Submucous myomas >15 mm, medical therapy may be considered to induce endometrial atrophy and reduce the size of the myoma, with insufficient evidence available to identify the best pharmacologic strategy.

Summary of evidence and discussion: In a study conducted by Fabio Parazzini et al., Danzol and GnRHa used as a medical treatment facilitates surgery, improving the long term results of myomectomy.

In incomplete myomectomy, GnRH analogue can be prescribed for 2–3 months to help migration of the intramural part of myoma before a second outpatient hysteroscopy is performed.

Q10. Is there a role of use of vasopressin in hysteroscopic myomectomy?

Draft recommendations: The existing literature confirms that with both intracervical and intralesional injection of dilute vasopressin, surgeons will be able to manage the bleeding and loss of fluid during myomectomy which leads to complete resection of myoma in one session.

Summary of evidence and discussion: In a study by Safoura Rouholamin et al. the mean time of myomectomy was 38.1 and 77.38 min in vasopressin and control groups, respectively ($p < 0.001$). The mean inflow volume was 2800 and 4100 in vasopressin and control groups, respectively ($p = 0.029$). The visual clarity score was 8.5 and 6.5 in the vasopressin and control groups, respectively ($p < 0.001$). In the vasopressin group, one vial (20 units) of vasopressin was diluted into 60 units of normal saline. 3 cc of vasopressin was injected in 3 points directly into the substance of myoma with the special needle for hysteroscopy.

Phiilips et al. described the intracervical injection of diluted (0.05 U/mL) with notable effect in complete resection of myoma, blood loss, distention fluid intravasation, and operative time during hysteroscopy, but also observed the intracervical injection of vasopressin might cause hypertension and bradycardia due to the possibility of injection into the uterine artery.

Q11. In asymptomatic submucous myoma, what is the current guidelines in management?

Draft recommendations:

- Expectant management is acceptable, but hysteroscopic myomectomy is recommended in patients where immediate fertility is not desired and in the presence of one asymptomatic submucous myoma <15 mm.
- If expectant management is done, clinical surveillance of symptoms and serial transvaginal pelvic ultrasounds is recommended to monitor growth of the myomas. When fertility is a priority and in the presence of one asymptomatic submucous myomas >15 mm, hysteroscopic myomectomy is recommended.

Summary of evidence and discussion: Only one RCT compared myomectomy to no surgery in women with myomas and infertility, included study of 181 women with a solitary myoma ≤4 cm in size and at least 1 year of infertility were randomized to surgery where they observed that clinical pregnancy rates were assessed based on location of myomas and the intervention. As there is fair evidence that hysteroscopic myomectomy for submucosal fibroids improves clinical pregnancy rates, when fertility is a priority, asymptomatic submucosal myomas need to ne resection out.

Q12. What are the complications of hysteroscopic myomectomy?

Draft recommendations: The incidence of complications in hysteroscopic myomectomy ranges from 0.8–2.6%. these include the following:

- Laceration of the cervix
- Uterine perforation
- Uterine bleeding
- Fluid Overload
- Air embolism

Summary of evidence and discussion: The use of saline and ringer lactate combined with bipolar current has minimal risk of complications of fluid overload and consequently, heart failure, but has eliminated the possibility of electrolyte complications.

Hysteroscopic myomectomy is associated with some late complications of intrauterine adhesions with an incidence of 1 to 13%, thus advocating a review of the uterine cavity especially in patients who desire to conceive, at

45 to 60 days postoperatively to review the uterine cavity and lysis of adhesions. These adhesions will be easily lysed with scissors or with the simple passage of the hysteroscope.

Despite the technique, a few myomas need second sitting, hence the importance of evaluating patient clinical condition and classification of fibroids for decisive data for knowledge and risk prevention due to safety concerns.

Q13. What are the clinical outcomes of hysteroscopic myomectomy?

Draft recommendations: Majority of patients experience significant improvement or resolution of symptoms related to fibroids, such as heavy bleeding, pelvic pain, and infertility with shorter recovery time after hysteroscopic myomectomy compared to open surgery. In women with infertility caused by submucosal fibroids, hysteroscopic myomectomy can significantly improve the chances of conception, involving minimal tissue damage to the uterus, preserving its structure and function.

Summary of evidence and discussion:

Abnormal uterine bleeding (AUB): The success rate of hysteroscopic myomectomy is as high as 70–99% with the size, number, and location of the fibroids as well as the surgeon's expertise and whether resection was complete or incomplete determining the success rate.

Fertility outcomes: Although submucosal fibroids are frequently implicated in patients with subfertility and hysteroscopic myomectomy is commonly recommended, the literature is currently inconsistent in this regard. The Practice Committee of the American Society for Reproductive Medicine (ASRM) created guidelines that explain the correlation between fertility and leiomyomas but the heterogeneity of the study populations, type, location, number and size of fibroids, and the inclusion and exclusion criteria led to difficulty drawing accurate conclusions to guide practice recommendations.

Final considerations: Hysteroscopic myomectomy is the most difficult and complex surgery among hysteroscopic surgeries, with a potential for serious risks and complications. Its performance can be safe and efficient for the treatment of intrauterine disease, especially being the best therapeutic option for submucous myomas.

Safety in myomectomy is at two distinct moments, in the preoperative evaluation and in the operative act. In the preoperative period, it consists of the hemodynamic evaluation of the patient, the knowledge of the desire for a future pregnancy, and the classification of the uterine fibroid.

8.3 HEMOSTASIS IN LAPAROSCOPIC MYOMECTOMY

Sanket Pisat, Suchita Pisat

Q1. What is the estimated blood loss and risk factors for intra operative hemorrhage in laparoscopic myomectomy surgery?

Draft recommendations:

- The incidence of blood loss in laparoscopic myomectomy is variable, ranging between 84 to 1,200 mL.
- The risk of bleeding increases with the following factors: Myoma size (8 cm or more), number of myomas (3 or more), location of myomas (intra mural myomas having more blood loss than subserous myomas), and increased surgical time due to other factors like BMI, surgeon skill, surgical adhesions etc.

Summary of evidence: A recently published systematic review and meta-analysis by Sleiman et al. in the Journal of Gynecology and Minimally Invasive Therapy investigating hemoglobin drop in women undergoing laparoscopic myomectomy reported an estimated intra-operative blood loss of 84–1200 mL, with increased risk of bleeding with myoma number and size. Increased blood loss was seen with more than 3 myomas removed. There was a linear relation of the size of the myoma with the intra operative blood loss. Intra mural myomas with a size of between 8 to 12 cm had a greater incidence of blood loss as compared to subserous myomas of similar size. When comparing blood transfusion, the study found that a surgery duration ≥240 min had a 4.8 times risk compared to <240 min. An operation time longer than 92 min was independently associated with more than two units drop in hemoglobin in another study.

Q2. What are the preoperative measures of decreasing blood loss during laparoscopic myomectomy, and how long should they be used?

Draft recommendations:

- Nonhormonal treatment options like tranexamic acid and NSAIDs, and systemic hormone therapy or contraceptives are offered for symptomatic relief from menorrhagia, but have no co relation with intra operative blood loss during surgery.
- Preoperative misoprostol may be used to reduce blood loss during open as well as laparoscopic myomectomy in a dose of 400 mcg 1 hour before surgery.
- Gonadotropin-releasing hormone (GnRH) may be used as a preoperative measure for large myomas in order to reduce the risk of hemorrhage. Usually with treatment for 6–8 weeks, reduction in fibroid size is seen along with a decrease in intra operative blood loss.

- Prolonged use of GnRH analogues is not recommended as they can obscure the tissue planes between fibroids and the myometrium, making enucleation difficult and increasing the chance of myoma recurrence.
- The effects of GnRH agonists wear off once the drug is discontinued, hence the timing of the operation close to the end of the treatment is necessary

Summary of evidence: As per a study published by Tanos et al. in Biomed Research International in 2018, systemic hormone therapy and contraceptives are generally the first line of treatment, especially for patients with heavy menstrual bleeding. Nonhormonal treatment options are also available, such as tranexamic acid and nonsteroidal anti-inflammatory agents. Another option is the use of Gonadotropin-releasing hormone (GnRH) or ulipristal acetate as a preoperative measure for large myomas in order to reduce the risk of hemorrhage. Usually with treatment for 6–8 weeks, fibroids shrink by 30–50%. The use of these agents should not exceed the 6–8 weeks, as they can obscure the tissue planes between fibroids and the myometrium, making enucleation difficult and increasing the chance of myoma recurrence. Once this agent is discontinued, myoma regrowth occurs; hence the timing of the operation close to the end of the treatment is necessary. Both the cost of the medication and the risk of cleavage plane lost must be weighed against the benefits when deciding whether or not to use them

Q3. What are the intra operative measures of reducing blood loss in laparoscopic myomectomy?

Draft recommendations:

- The use of vasopressin significantly reduces the intra operative blood loss in laparoscopic myomectomy and is recommended unless specifically contra indicated due to medical reasons like known hypersensitivity.
- Ligation of the uterine arteries at the origin reduces the intra operative blood loss, but may be associated with increased operative time.
- Though not used routinely, there is *low-quality* evidence that bupivacaine plus epinephrine, tranexamic acid, a peri-cervical tourniquet or a tourniquet tied round both cervix and infundibulopelvic ligament may reduce bleeding during myomectomy.

Summary of recommendations: A Cochrane review published by Kongnyuy EJ et al. in 2014 stated that there is *moderate-quality* evidence that misoprostol or vasopressin may reduce bleeding during myomectomy. The reviewers found significant reductions in the need for blood transfusion, in open myomectomy with vasopressin, tourniquet tied round the cervix, tourniquet tied round both cervix and infundibulopelvic ligament but no evidence of any change on the need for blood transfusion with misoprostol, oxytocin, tranexamic acid, ascorbic acid, loop ligation of the myoma pseudo-capsule and a fibrin sealant patch

Q4. What is the effective dose of vasopressin for reducing blood loss in laparoscopic myomectomy, with minimum systemic side effects?

Draft recommendations:

1. The minimum concentration of vasopressin for achieving acceptable hemostasis must be used in surgery.
2. A dose of 0.1 IU/mL (1 ampoule of 20 units vasopressin diluted in 200 mL NS) to 0.05 IU/mL (1 ampoule of 20 units vasopressin diluted in 400 mL NS) gives comparable outcomes to higher concentrations like 0.2 IU/mL and is recommended for optimizing surgical hemostasis, while minimizing potential side effects

Summary of recommendation: The VALENTINE trial by Soo Jin Park et al. in 2024 is the first randomized controlled pilot trial to evaluate the efficacy and safety of diluted concentrations of vasopressin at the same infusion volume in reducing blood loss during robotic assisted laparoscopic myomectomy (RALM). This trial comparing the hemostatic effect and safety of three different concentrations of vasopressin (0.2 IU/mL, 0.1 IU/mL, and 0.05 IU/mL) in a volume of 100 mL of normal saline showed comparable outcomes among the three different concentrations. However, the highest concentration of vasopressin (0.2 IU/mL) was associated with a 15.4% incidence of unnecessary intraoperative hypertension, suggesting that dilution of vasopressin to 0.05 IU/mL may be both effective and safe for hemostasis during RALM

Q5. What are the side effects/hazards of using vasopressin during laparoscopic myomectomy?

Draft recommendations:

- Vasopressin can cause generalized hypotension, hypertension, tachycardia, bradycardia, peripheral pulselessness with an unrecordable SPO_2 due to peripheral vasospasm, cardiac arrest, cardiac arrhythmias, myocardial infarction and pulmonary edema after injection.
- The effects are usually seen within 2 to 3 minutes of injection, which may be due to inadvertent intravascular injection.
- Side effects may be seen up to 10 minutes of injection, usually due to systemic absorption of the drug rather than inadvertent intravascular injection.
- Typically, these effects are transient and hemodynamic parameters return to normal within 15 to 25 minutes of injection.

Summary of recommendation: A review article by Eu Jin Lee et al. in the BMJ in 2022 states that vasopressin can cause general hypotension and severe vasoconstriction within 2 or 3 min when vasopressin is injected into the muscular layer of the uterus. Typically, these changes return to normal after 15–25 min, but they can also have a fatal effect on the patient. Their severe complications mainly affect cardiopulmonary function, such as sudden cardiac arrest starting with bradycardia or acrotism, pulmonary edema and myocardial infarction

Q6. How can the hazards of using vasoconstrictive agents during laparoscopic myomectomy be minimized?

Draft recommendations:

- Using the minimum acceptable concentration of vasopressin solution reduces the potential systemic side effects as compared to higher concentrations.
- The use of a laparoscopic device to detect inadvertent intravascular puncture minimizes the possibility of systemic injection of vasopressin, though it does not completely negate the possibility of side effects.
- Vasopressin should be avoided in patients with a high likelihood of complications like known hypersensitivity to the drug, uncontrolled hypertension and cardiac diseases.

Summary of recommendations: The VALENTINE trial, as previously stated, recommends a dose of 0.5 to 1 IU/mL as a safe dose for infiltration during laparoscopic myomectomy. As per a recent publication by Rabie S et al. in the Indian journal of anesthesia in 2021, avoiding the intravascular injection and avoiding the drug in those with cardiovascular diseases, those with a history of smoking and careful observations of the heart rate, blood pressure, and ECG during and after the vasopressin injection in addition to the proper selection of patients reduces the incidence of severe complications. Pisat, S and van Herendael B, published the use of an innovative device for detecting inadvertent intravascular puncture before laparoscopic injection of vasopressin solution into the myoma, significantly reducing the possibility of hemodynamic fluctuations after injection. Further publications by Jain N et al. highlighted the role of this device in laparoscopic myomectomy

Q7. How effective is laparoscopic uterine artery ligation at origin in reducing intra operative hemorrhage during laparoscopic myomectomy, and in which cases should it be used?

Draft recommendations:

- In smaller fibroids (single myoma, subserous in location, less than 8 cm in size), vasopressin provides acceptable control of bleeding intra operatively. In these cases, uterine artery occlusion has only a modest effect on the mean reduction of blood loss and reduction of blood transfusion, and may not have significant clinical benefit.

- In large (more than 8 cm), multiple (more than 3) and deep (intramural) myomas, the addition of uterine artery ligation reduces the intra operative blood loss by up to 50 percent, and is recommended.
- Factors such as surgeon skill in performing safe surgical dissection to reach the uterine artery, and the increase in operative time must be considered before deciding to use this approach.

Summary of recommendation: An article published by Bedaiwy M in Fertil Steril in 2019 states that the absolute risk of blood transfusion reduction was only 7.2% in the uterine artery occlusion myomectomy group, with a mean difference of 0.60 g/dL in the change in hemoglobin values compared with control subjects. The modest effect of uterine artery occlusion on the primary outcomes (mean reduction of blood loss by only 103 mL and absolute risk reduction of blood transfusion by 7.2%) casts some doubt on the practical clinical benefit and utility of this radical intervention, particularly when uterine artery occlusion is bilateral and permanent.

Hiratsuka et al. in 2022, in the European journal of Obs and Gyne stated that intraoperative blood loss volume was decreased by approximately half with the addition of temporary uterine artery ligation(but the operation time was longer.

Liu et al. in Fertil Steril 2011, stated that the procedure can be performed in under 10 minutes by an experienced gynecologist, has remarkably decreased blood loss in laparoscopic myomectomy, and it has expanded the application of LM greatly, such as the large, multiple, and deep myomas located in the uterus.

Q8. Is there a place for reversible ligation of the uterine artery at its origin in patients desirous of future fertility?

Draft recommendations:

- It is unclear whether permanent bilateral uterine artery occlusion causes infertility or perinatal complications in patients desirous of fertility such as increased abortion rate and preterm delivery.
- Laparoscopic transient uterine artery ligation does not produce any appreciable adverse effect on fertility, and can safely be performed in patients desirous of fertility.
- Titanium clips for are not designed for removal after insertion, and the removal procedure might cause additional problems, such as vessel injury. Temporary uterine artery ligation with a slip knot using a multifilament suture material allows easy reversal of the ligation at the end of surgery.

Summary of recommendation: Hiratsuka et al. in 2022, in the European Journal of Obs and Gyne stated that is unclear whether permanent bilateral uterine artery occlusion causes infertility or perinatal complications in patients desirous of fertility such as increased abortion rate and preterm delivery. They also stated that Titanium clips for are not designed for removal after insertion, and the removal procedure might cause additional problems, such as vessel injury. Temporary uterine artery ligation with a slip knot using a multifilament suture material allows easy reversal of the ligation at the end of surgery. Liu et al. in Fertil Steril 2011, stated that Laparoscopic transient uterine artery ligation does not produce any appreciable adverse effect on fertility, and can safely be performed in patients desirous of fertility. Pisat S et al. in 2020 and Desai P et al. in 2022 have described the use of a laparoscopic 'Shoelace' knot for reversible uterine artery ligation at its origin in indicated cases.

8.4 LAPAROSCOPIC MYOMECTOMY

Soumil Trivedi, Prakash Trivedi, Kaustav Kar

Q1. What are the indications for laparoscopic myomectomy?

Draft recommendations:

- Laparoscopic myomectomy is indicated for symptomatic uterine fibroids causing heavy menstrual bleeding, pelvic pain, pressure symptoms, infertility, or recurrent pregnancy loss. It is also considered for fibroids that are rapidly growing, causing urinary or bowel dysfunction.
- Indications for a laparoscopic myomectomy are continuously expanding and not limited by size, number or location with appropriate patient selection, surgeon's skills and requisite technology and infrastructure.
- Fibroids more than 8 cm in size, more than 4 in number and low isthmo-cervical or other oddly located fibroids may pose challenges for an inexperienced surgeon.
- Laparoscopic myomectomy may be indicated in cases of subfertility for large submucous or cavity distorting fibroids of >4 cm size, intramural fibroids >5 cm or even subserous fibroids >7 cm.

Summary of evidence: The maximum size for laparoscopic myomectomy is generally 8–10 cm, with a limit of four fibroids being commonly accepted based on various clinical studies. This limitation is due to the technical challenges posed by larger or more numerous fibroids, which may increase the risk of complications such as bleeding and conversion to open surgery. Holub et al. (2007) and Advincula et al., (2004) support these size and number thresholds. The presence of non-cavity-distorting intramural fibroids is associated with adverse pregnancy outcomes in women undergoing IVF treatment (Sunkara et al., 2010).

Q2. What preoperative evaluations are essential before performing a laparoscopic myomectomy?

Draft recommendations:

- Preoperative evaluations include a detailed medical history, physical examination, and imaging with pelvic ultrasound or MRI to assess the size, number, and location of fibroids. Complete blood count and coagulation profile, are necessary to evaluate anemia and bleeding risk. Endometrial sampling may be indicated in high-risk patients to exclude malignancy.
- MRI may be recommended in multiple fibroids for accurate mapping, presence of any degenerations and in rapidly growing fibroids, post-menopausal increase in size of fibroids to rule out suspicion of undiagnosed malignancy.
- Serum lactate dehydrogenase (LDH) especially LDH isoenzyme 3 may be considered to establish a revised PREoperative Sarcoma Score (rPRESS) concerning leiomyosarcoma

Summary of evidence: MRI is particularly useful in assessing the exact location and size of fibroids, especially when multiple fibroids are present. A study by Dueholm et al., (2001) showed that MRI provides superior accuracy compared to transvaginal ultrasonography in fibroid mapping. Preoperative evaluations play a crucial role in surgical planning and improving outcomes. Utility of rPRESS score given by Nagai et al., 2015.

Q3. What are the benefits of laparoscopic myomectomy compared to open myomectomy?

Draft recommendations: It is preferrable to have a minimal invasive approach to myomectomy as it offers benefits such as smaller incisions, reduced postoperative pain, faster recovery, shorter hospital stays, and a lower risk of wound infections and adhesions. This also results in less blood loss and better cosmetic outcomes compared to open myomectomy.

Summary of evidence: Meta-analyses comparing laparoscopic to open myomectomy demonstrate fewer postoperative complications and shorter recovery times. Jin et al., (2009) showed that laparoscopic myomectomy is associated with a lower risk of complications (OR 0.47, 95% CI 0.26 to 0.85) compared to open myomectomy, making it the preferred approach when feasible.

Q4. What are the potential risks and complications of laparoscopic myomectomy?

Answer: Risks include bleeding, infection, injury to surrounding organs (bladder, bowel, ureters), adhesion formation, and recurrence of fibroids. There is also a possibility of conversion to open surgery if complications arise or if the fibroids are too large or numerous for safe laparoscopic removal.

Summary of evidence: Studies, such as those by Miller and Wechter (2015), indicate that the complication rate for laparoscopic myomectomy is low but may include injury to adjacent organs and significant bleeding, particularly with larger fibroids. Adhesion formation remains a concern, although less frequent than with open surgery .

Q5. What is the role of preoperative medical therapy in laparoscopic myomectomy?

Draft recommendations: Medical modalities such as GnRH agonists and antagonists shrink fibroids and reduce vascularity but have hypoestrogenic side effects; ulipristal acetate also reduces fibroid size with fewer side effects, while mifepristone reduces fibroid volume and softens tissue with a milder side-effect profile but requires endometrial monitoring.

Surgical challenges due to preoperative therapy:

- *Loss of planes:* Medical management of fibroids with GnRH analogues or SPRMs can reduce fibroid size and symptoms, but it may also obscure surgical planes, making myomectomy more challenging. The resulting shrinkage and fibrosis can increase the risk of incomplete removal, surgical complications, and longer operative times. (Talulikar et al., 2012).
- *Myoma migration:* Shrinkage of fibroids due to preoperative therapy especially with SPRMs can cause their position to shift within the uterus, altering the surgical approach. In some cases, this migration can improve access to deeper fibroids, aiding the surgeon in a more straightforward removal.

Summary of evidence:

- *GnRH analog therapy:* According to a Cochrane review by Lethaby et al., (2002), GnRH analogs can reduce fibroid size by up to 50%, significantly reducing intraoperative blood loss and improving the ease of fibroid removal. However, GnRH therapy causes menopausal-like side effects such as hot flashes, bone loss, and mood disturbances, limiting its use to short durations before surgery. It can also cause loss of surgical planes (Talulikar et al., 2012).
- *Ulipristal acetate:* A randomized controlled trial by Donnez et al. (2012) demonstrated that ulipristal acetate effectively reduces fibroid size and controls symptoms of heavy menstrual bleeding, with a more favorable side-effect profile compared to GnRH agonists. The reduction in fibroid size by 20–50% helps improve surgical conditions, and its use is typically limited to 3 months preoperatively. It has been associated with rare but serious cases of liver injury, including hepatic failure. Due to these risks, regulatory bodies like the European Medicines Agency (EMA) have recommended regular monitoring of liver function tests (LFTs) during treatment. The medication is contraindicated in patients with existing

liver conditions, and treatment should be discontinued if liver function deteriorates. These precautions are crucial to prevent severe liver damage, as reported cases have led to liver transplantation in some instances.

- *Mifepristone:* Studies (Fiscella et al., 2006) have shown that mifepristone reduces fibroid volume by 30–50%, leading to improved surgical outcomes by decreasing fibroid size, softening fibroid consistency, and reducing intraoperative blood loss. Mifepristone is well-tolerated, but endometrial monitoring is required due to potential changes in the endometrium, such as hyperplasia.

Q6. What are the long-term outcomes of laparoscopic myomectomy in terms of fibroid recurrence and fertility?

Answer: Long-term outcomes indicate that fibroid recurrence rates can reach 27% over five years. However, laparoscopic myomectomy improves fertility outcomes, with pregnancy rates comparable to those following open myomectomy. Uterine rupture during pregnancy is a rare complication, provided the uterine defect is closed appropriately, often with a double-layer technique.

Summary of evidence: A meta-analysis by Tanos et al. (2023) found that laparoscopic myomectomy results in improved fertility outcomes with low complication rates during subsequent pregnancies. Proper uterine closure techniques, particularly two-layer suturing, minimize the risk of uterine rupture .

Q7. What are the indications for converting a laparoscopic myomectomy to an open procedure?

Answer: Conversion to open surgery may be necessary in cases of uncontrollable bleeding, extensive adhesions, or if fibroids are too large or numerous for safe removal laparoscopically. Other reasons include poor visualization or complications arising during the procedure.

Summary of evidence: Conversion rates are typically low in experienced hands. Pritts et al. (2017) found that the most common reasons for conversion include uncontrolled bleeding and poor anatomical visualization, often related to the size or number of fibroids.

Q8. What are the indications where an open procedure is preferred over a laparoscopy?

Draft recommendations: Open myomectomy is preferred over laparoscopic myomectomy in the following cases:

- *Large fibroids:* Typically, fibroids larger than 10–12 cm in diameter may be better suited for open surgery due to limited space for instrument manoeuvring in laparoscopy and the potential for incomplete removal, especially in a resource-poor setting or in case of an inexperienced surgeon.

- *Multiple fibroids:* When more than 5 fibroids are present, the complexity of removal increases, making open surgery a safer and more effective option in some cases, again this too is highly dependent on surgeon's skills and tools.
- *Deep intramural fibroids:* Fibroids deeply embedded in the uterine wall can pose challenges for laparoscopic removal, with a higher risk of incomplete excision and significant bleeding.
- *Pelvic adhesions:* Extensive adhesions due to previous surgeries or conditions like endometriosis can obstruct visualization and increase the risk of injury to surrounding organs during laparoscopy.
- *Complex fibroid locations:* Fibroids located in challenging areas near vital structures such as the bladder, bowel, ureters or major blood vessels may be more safely removed through an open approach.
- *Uncontrolled bleeding disorders:* Patients with uncontrolled bleeding disorders are at increased risk of significant intraoperative and postoperative bleeding, making laparoscopic procedures less safe. *Suspected malignancy:* Laparoscopic myomectomy is contraindicated in patients with suspected uterine malignancy, such as leiomyosarcoma, due to the risk of spreading cancerous cells during tissue manipulation and morcellation.
- *Severe cardio-respiratory disoreders:* Laparoscopic myomectomy which usually requires employing general anesthesia with intubation, creation of pneumoperitoneum and use of trendelenburg position may exacerbate cardio-respiratory embarrassment making open surgery the preferred option.

Consideration of surgeon expertise, equipment, and infrastructure: While these are common indications for open myomectomy, the choice between an open or laparoscopic approach depends significantly on the surgeon's expertise, available equipment, and the infrastructure of the facility. Surgeons with advanced laparoscopic skills, specialized tools (e.g., morcellators, high-definition laparoscopic cameras), and adequate support systems may successfully perform laparoscopic myomectomy even in more complex cases. On the other hand, in facilities lacking these resources, or when the surgeon has limited laparoscopic experience, open surgery may provide better safety and outcomes.

Summary of evidence: A systematic review was performed on published randomized controlled trials on laparoscopic versus open myomectomy were assessed on operative parameters and outcomes. Six studies and 576 patients were studied by Chu Jin 2009 it showed that laparoscopic myomectomy, when performed by specialized surgeons on selected patients, resulted in less hemoglobin drop, reduced blood loss, faster recovery, less postoperative pain, and fewer complications compared to open surgery, though it takes longer. Major complications, pregnancy outcomes, and recurrence rates are similar in both approaches, making laparoscopy a better option overall.

Q9. What are the different types of laparoscopic containment devices/ systems available for morcellation in laparoscopic myomectomy, and what are their advantages and disadvantages?

Answer: Containment devices include specialized containment bags, some may not be FDA approved, all designed to prevent tissue spillage during morcellation. These devices reduce the risk of spreading fibroid tissue or undetected malignancies. Tissue retrieval techniques are discussed under a separate section.

Summary of evidence: Cohen et al., (2016) emphasized the importance of containment systems during morcellation to prevent the inadvertent spread of malignancies such as leiomyosarcoma. The FDA has recommended the use of containment systems in all morcellation procedures.

Q10. What are the advantages of barbed sutures over traditional sutures?

Summary of evidence: Barbed sutures offer several advantages over traditional sutures in laparoscopic myomectomy:

- *No need for knot tying:* Barbed sutures self-anchor in tissue, eliminating the need for knot tying, which can simplify and expedite the suturing process. (Greenberg, 2013)
- *Even distribution of tension:* Provides consistent tension along the suture line, which can improve wound closure and healing.
- *Reduced operative time:* Faster suturing process can reduce overall operative time, which may decrease anesthesia duration and associated risks. (Einarsson, 2014)
- *Improved hemostasis:* Barbed sutures can enhance hemostasis by providing better tissue approximation, which helps reduce intraoperative bleeding (Rosen, 2015)

Q11. What are the Challenges one may encounter at various steps of laparoscopic myomectomy with potential solutions?

Sr. No	Challenges	Solutions
1.	Preoperative evaluation and surgical planning	• An MRI may be indicated in multiple fibroids for accurate mapping, very large fibroid, rapidly growing fibroids, hypervascular fibroids, fibroids with suspicion of malignant changes • LDH especially, isoenzyme Type 3 may be indicated in suspicion of leiomyosarcoma with limited benefit, as it can often be deranged in degenerated fibroids and patients who have undergone prolonged medical therapy with drugs like ulipristal acetate
2.	Incision planning	• The choice of vertical or horizontal incision is usually based on surgeon's preference and method adopted for suturing namely contralateral or ipsilateral • Horizontal incision usually does not cut through the uterine vasculature and are sometimes favourable to reduce bleeding • In large fibroids with myometrium stretched over the myoma, an elliptical incision may be preferred to aid quick enucleation, reduction of dead space, and make suturing efficient
3.	Hemostatic measures	• Preoperative use of per-rectal misoprostol and IV trenaxamic acid have been shown to reduce blood loss • Retroperitoneal dissection and laparoscopic uterine artery ligation (LUAL) at the origin using temporary measures like shoelace knot or hemo-clips may be considered in very large, multiple, hypervascular fibroids and is not shown to affect fertility outcomes • Use of dilute vasopression helps in reducing bloodloss, repeat instillation may be considered for multiple fibroids but for solitary large fibroids it may be preferrable to re-inject in the uterine musculature rather than the myoma-myometrial junction • Hemostatic measures in laparoscopic myomectomy are covered in details in section 8.3
4.	Large size	• Usually, the primary port is placed 8-10 cm above the palpable fundal edge and corresponding secondary ports may need to be taken slightly higher • Use of additional secondary ports may sometimes be useful for myoma-manipulation with a myoma-spiral. In very large-to-heavy fibroids use of two myoma -spirals or a 10 mm myoma spiral may be considered
5.	Multiple Fibroids	• In multiple fibroids based on the mapping it is preferrable to remove as many myomas as possible from a single incision but may not always be feasible. If multiple incisions are taken it is preferrable to suture one defect and then proceed to the next, to reduce bleeding

Contd...

Contd…

Sr. No	***Challenges***	***Solutions***
		• To minimize losing the fibroids in the peritoneal cavity after enucleation, proper fibroid count must be maintained and optional stringing up of especially small fibroids with a suture can be considered. However, stringing up of multiple large fibroids may pose a difficulty in manipulation of the fibroids into containment systems
6.	Odd locations	• In low isthmic or cervical fibroid spreading laterally, it may be preferrable to take a vertical incision to safeguard vital structures • In broad ligament fibroids, incision is usually based on the bulge but a posterior incision over the stretched peritoneum when feasible is preferrable as it obviates the need of suturing and provides natural drainage
7.	Safe-guarding vital structures	• In case of anatomical distortion due to large, oddly situated or multiple fibroids, use of ureteric stents, especially illuminated or cystoscopy ureteric ICG dye instillation to visualize the ureters and safeguard them is a preferable option. Ureterolysis may also be required in some fibroids with extension into the lateral pelvic wall • Remaining intracapsular while enucleation preserving the pseudocapsule adds to safety and also preserves the neurovascular bundle which helps in healing
8.	Suturing	• Whenever the dead space following fibroid enucleation is large with lot of redundant myometrium, layered closure completely obliterating the dead space is imperative for proper healing, hemostasis and adhesion prevention • Occasionally, box sutures or horizontal mattress sutures may be taken to appose the edges and reach the base of the defect before layered closure
9.	Tissue retrieval	• Covered in details in section 8.5 on tissue retrieval
10.	Adhesion prevention	• Adhering to micro-surgical principles with good hemostasis and tissue approximation helps in preventing adhesions • When using barbed sutures, taking baseball stitches for the outermost layer helps in reducing adhesions and also complications like subacute bowel obstruction • Use of adhesion prevention barriers like interceed etc. may be helpful • *Pharmacological methods:* NSAIDs (Ibuprofen, Ketorolac), corticosteroids (Dexamethasone, Methylprednisolone), fibrinolytic agents (tPA [Activase]), anti-fibrotic agents (Pirfenidone [Esbriet]), and hyaluronic acid-based solutions (Intergel, Seprafilm [Hyalobarrier]) • *Barrier methods:* Seprafilm (Hyalobarrier), Interceed (Oxidized Regenerated Cellulose), Adept (Icodextrin), and Gore-Tex surgical membranes

Research gap: Surgical steps and techniques followed during laparoscopic myomectomy may vary depending on individual surgeon preferences, patient-specific factors, and the complexity of the case. While a structured approach can guide key aspects of the procedure, the evolving nature of surgical innovation and advancements in technology mean that a one-size-fits-all protocol may not be feasible. Therefore, adapting the surgical plan to the patient's unique anatomy, fibroid characteristics, and the surgeon's expertise is crucial. A standardized approach to laparoscopic myomectomy remains difficult to establish, but adherence to evidence-based practices and continuous training will ensure the best outcomes.

8.5 TISSUE RETRIEVAL—CHALLENGES AND OPTIONS

Soumil Trivedi, Prakash Trivedi, Kaustav Kar

Q1. What are the main tissue retrieval techniques used in laparoscopic myomectomy or hysterectomy done for fibroids?

The various tissue retrieval techniques include:

a. Power morcellation
b. Manual morcellation
c. Laparotomy
d. Minilaparotomy
e. Minilaparotomy with manual morcellation
f. Natural orifice specimen extraction (NOSE)
g. Endo-bag retrieval

Q2. Why did electromechanical (power) morcellation come into disrepute and under scrutiny? What are the chances of accidental power-morcellation of undiagnosed leiomyosarcoma?

Summary of evidence: Electromechanical (power) morcellation came under scrutiny and disrepute primarily due to concerns about its potential to spread undiagnosed malignant tissues, such as leiomyosarcoma, during laparoscopic procedures. In 2014, the U.S. Food and Drug Administration (FDA) issued a safety communication after reviewing reports of unsuspected uterine sarcomas being disseminated by power morcellators used during fibroid removal surgeries, significantly worsening patient outcomes.

Studies indicated that approximately 1 in 350 women undergoing fibroid removal may have an undiagnosed uterine sarcoma, and morcellation could inadvertently spread cancerous cells throughout the abdomen and pelvis, reducing survival rates. Following this, the FDA recommended against using power morcellators in most hysterectomy and myomectomy cases for fibroids, leading to a dramatic reduction in their use and the development of safer alternatives like contained morcellation. In a 2015 meta-analysis by Pritts et al., the estimated rate of leiomyosarcoma was 0.51 per 1,000 procedures or approximately 1 in 2,000; restricting the meta-analysis to the 64 prospective studies resulted in a substantially lower estimate of 0.12 leiomyosarcomas per 1,000 procedures or approximately 1 leiomyosarcoma per 8,300 surgeries.

Q3. How should patients be evaluated pre-operatively for laparoscopic myomectomy?

Draft recommendations: Conduct a comprehensive evaluation including:

- Detailed medical history and physical examination
- Imaging studies (ultrasound, doppler study, MRI) to assess fibroid characteristics
- Evaluation of risk factors for malignancy (e.g., age, family history, symptoms)- revised PREoperative Sarcoma Score (rPRESS)
- Discussion of surgical options and associated risks with the patient

Summary of evidence: It would be ideal to be able to predict preoperatively whether a presumed fibroid is actually a malignancy. Unfortunately, we do not have reliable ways to determine this. Demographic factors such as age or rapid tumor growth are not helpful, especially because occult malignancy may be present in women in their 20s and 30s.

Preoperative imaging shows promise, but its clinical utility is yet to be determined. A 2002 study by Hata et al. shows that there was no significant difference in the resistive index (RI) between uterine leiomyomas and sarcomas. However, the peak systolic velocity (PSV) was significantly higher in uterine sarcomas (median 61.6 cm/s) compared to leiomyomas (median 21.6 cm/s) ($p < 0.05$). A PSV cut-off of 41.0 cm/s detected uterine sarcomas with 80.0% accuracy and a 2.4% false-positive rate. Two preliminary studies using MRI with lactate dehydrogenase (LDH) isoenzyme 3 measurements or with diffusion-weighted imaging demonstrated promising results (Goto et al., 2002) but more research is needed before recommending routine MRIs before all surgeries for presumed leiomyomas. Nagai's revised PREoperative Sarcoma Score (rPRESS) offers a predictive tool to assess malignancy risk, integrating factors like patient age, serum Lactate Dehydrogenase Isoenzyme 3 and imaging findings. The cost of such a measure would be significant and the chance of false-positive results is high, given the rarity of these conditions.

Q4. What factors should be considered when selecting a tissue retrieval technique?

Draft recommendations: When selecting a tissue retrieval technique, several key factors should be considered like size and number of specimens, oncological risk, safety concerns, patient factors, preferences, financial considerations, surgeon expertise and equipment availability

Summary of evidence: When selecting a tissue retrieval technique for myomectomy or hysterectomy, evidence-based factors include: larger or multiple fibroids often require morcellation; contained morcellation or en bloc resection is recommended if malignancy is suspected to prevent tissue dissemination; safety concerns favor contained techniques for reducing infection risk; patient factors like body habitus can influence method choice; surgeon expertise with specific techniques affects outcomes; equipment availability is essential for advanced methods; patient preferences regarding cosmetic outcomes are significant; and cost considerations are crucial, especially in resource-limited settings.

Q5. What are containment systems and in-bag morcellation, and how does it enhance safety?

Containment systems enhance safety due to following factors:

- Prevents tissue dissemination
- Minimizes organ injury
- Oncological safety
- Reduces postoperative complications

Summary of evidence: Containment systems are specialized surgical devices used in laparoscopic procedures to enclose tissues, such as uterine fibroids, during morcellation, enhancing safety through several evidence-based mechanisms. First, they prevent tissue dissemination by keeping tissues enclosed, which minimizes the risk of spreading benign or malignant cells and reduces complications like parasitic myomas or undetected cancers, such as leiomyosarcoma. Second, these systems minimize organ injury by acting as a barrier between the morcellator and surrounding organs, thereby reducing the risk of accidental injury to structures like the bowel or bladder. In instances where malignancy is a concern, containment systems provide oncological safety by preventing the dissemination of cancerous tissue during morcellation. Finally, containing tissue helps reduce postoperative complications related to tissue left in the abdominal cavity, such as adhesions and infections. Residual tissue may result in recurrence of fibroids, necessitating further surgeries. Additionally, larger tissue fragments may require larger incisions, increasing the risk of incisional hernia, and challenges in retrieval can prolong operating time, raising overall surgical risks.

Overall, containment systems significantly enhance the safety of tissue retrieval procedures by addressing critical risks associated with morcellation.

Q6. Does use of containment systems completely eliminate the risk of tissue dissemination, leiomyomatosis or upstaging of undiagnosed malignancies?

No, the use of containment systems *does not completely eliminate* the risk of tissue dissemination, leiomyomatosis, or upstaging of undiagnosed malignancies, but it *significantly reduces these risks* compared to uncontained morcellation.

Summary of evidence:

Reasons for continued risk:

1. *Inherent limitations of the system:* Small leaks or accidental breaches in the containment bag during the procedure can still result in tissue spillage.
2. *Tissue handling errors:* Especially in cases of *large fibroids* or *complex tissue morphology.*
3. *Undiagnosed malignancies:* In cases where a malignancy such as *leiomyosarcoma* is undiagnosed preoperatively, even with containment systems, some cancerous cells may escape or be upstaged if not completely confined. The malignancy could also spread before the bag is deployed or if manipulation is done outside the bag.
4. *Risk of leiomyomatosis: Benign metastasizing leiomyomatosis,* where benign fibroid fragments spread and implant in other parts of the abdomen, can still occur, although the risk is much lower when containment systems are used.

Q7. What safety measures should be taken to minimize the risk of tissue dissemination?

Draft recommendations: Following safety measures can be implemented:

- Use containment systems for morcellation
- Perform thorough inspection of the abdominal cavity for any tissue fragments
- Handle tissues carefully to prevent spillage
- At the end of morcellation, a thorough lavage is questionable
- Consider pre-operative endometrial sampling for patients at risk of malignancy

Q8. What are the potential complications of tissue retrieval in laparoscopic myomectomy?

Summary of evidence: Laparoscopic morcellation has important drawbacks that include the risk of severe trauma, tissue disruption that makes pathologic diagnosis more difficult, and dispersion of the morcellated tissue throughout the abdominal cavity. Less-serious consequences of tissue dispersion include cases of endometriosis and adenomyosis as well as leiomyomatosis, which are estimated to occur in 0.9% of patients having laparoscopic morcellation. A more serious consequence is dissemination of occult malignancy.

Q9. What are the different types of laparoscopic containment devices/ systems available for morcellation in laparoscopic myomectomy, and what are their advantages and disadvantages?

Several types of laparoscopic containment devices and systems are available for morcellation in laparoscopic myomectomy to prevent tissue dissemination. These include specialized commercially available US FDA approved or non-approved but widely used containment bags and indigenous innovations like modified Urobag systems, the use of surgical gloves ,etc. Here are their advantages and disadvantages:

- *Advantages:*
  - *High containment:* Provides robust containment of tissue fragments, significantly reducing the risk of spreading benign or malignant cells.
  - *Enhanced safety:* Minimizes the risk of parasitic fibroid formation and malignant cell dissemination within the abdominal cavity.
  - *Designed for procedure:* Specifically created for morcellation, making them user-friendly and efficient.
- *Disadvantages:*
  - *Increased complexity:* May add complexity to the procedure and require additional surgical skills.
  - *Longer operative time:* Can increase the duration of the surgery.
  - *Higher cost:* More expensive compared to makeshift containment methods.

Q10. How do various tissue retrieval techniques compare in terms of advantages, disadvantages, ideal case use?

Tissue retrieval techniques in laparoscopic myomectomy:

Technique	*Procedure*	*Advantages*	*Disadvantages*	*Ideal case scenario uses*
Mini-laparotomy	A small incision (mini-laparotomy) is made in the abdomen to manually remove the fibroid intact without debulking	Direct visualization and removal of fibroids	• Larger incision compared to other laparoscopic methods. • Increased wound related complications like infection, hernia etc.	Suitable for small fibroids up to 6 cm

Contd…

Contd…

Technique	***Procedure***	***Advantages***	***Disadvantages***	***Ideal case scenario uses***
Mini-lap with manual morcellation	A small incision is made in the abdomen and manual debulking with scalpel or scissors is done to cut the fibroid into smaller pieces	Allows removal of large fibroids through small incisions	• Risk of tissue dissemination and potential spread of undiagnosed malignancy. • Increased wound related complications like infection, hernia etc.	Suitable for larger fibroids where intact removal is impractical
Vaginal extraction (NOSE)	The fibroid or uterus with fibroid(s) is delivered through the vaginal canal, either directly or after being morcellated or debulked.	No abdominal incision required	Limited to smaller fibroids and requires vaginal access	Suitable for cases in which the vagina is opened intentionally like in hysterectomy or accidentally in low cervical fibroids
Endo-bag retrieval with manual morcellation	The fibroid is placed in a containment bag within the abdominal cavity before morcellation	Reduces risk of tissue dis-semination	May be time-consuming and technically challenging	Suitable for large or degenerated fibroids or fibroids with high suspicion of malignancy
Colpotomy	An incision is made in the vaginal wall (colpotomy) to allow removal of the fibroid	No abdominal incision and can be combined with vaginal myomectomy	Potential for pelvic floor dysfunction and longer recovery	Suitable for moderate to even large fibroids with cruciate or vertical colpotomy but can cause adhesions and dyspareunia

Contd…

Contd...

Technique	*Procedure*	*Advantages*	*Disadvantages*	*Ideal Case scenario uses*
Contained power morcellation	A powered morcellator is used within a containment bag to cut the fibroid into smaller pieces for removal. Power morcellation when employed, should preferably be done in a contained fashion	Efficient removal of large fibroids	High cost and risk of equipment-related complications	Suitable for all fibroids but can increase the operating time due to additional maneuvers required and loss of assistance

Research gaps:

1. *Long-term outcomes and complications:*
   - *Gap:* Limited longitudinal studies comparing the long-term outcomes and complications associated with different tissue retrieval techniques.
   - *Implication:* Understanding the long-term impacts is crucial for informed decision-making and improving patient care.
2. *Risk of tissue dissemination and malignancy:*
   - *Gap:* Insufficient data on the incidence of tissue dissemination and malignancy spread, particularly with morcellation techniques.
   - *Implication:* More research is needed to develop safer morcellation methods and protocols to minimize these risks.
3. *Comparative effectiveness of retrieval methods:*
   - *Gap:* Lack of comprehensive comparative studies evaluating the effectiveness, safety, and patient outcomes of various tissue retrieval techniques.
   - *Implication:* Direct comparisons can guide clinicians in selecting the most appropriate technique for different clinical scenarios.
4. *Technological innovations and improvements:*
   - *Gap:* Need for innovation in morcellation technology to enhance safety and efficiency.
   - *Implication:* Advances could lead to improved patient outcomes and reduced complication rates.

5. *Training and skill development:*
   - *Gap:* Limited research on the impact of surgeon experience and training on the outcomes of different tissue retrieval methods.
   - *Implication:* Standardized training protocols could improve the safety and effectiveness of laparoscopic myomectomy.
6. *Patient selection criteria:*
   - *Gap*: Inadequate evidence to establish clear guidelines on patient selection for different tissue retrieval techniques.
   - *Implication:* More precise criteria can help tailor the approach to individual patient needs, improving outcomes and reducing risks.
7. *Cost-effectiveness analysis:*
   - *Gap:* Few studies evaluating the cost-effectiveness of different tissue retrieval techniques in laparoscopic myomectomy.
   - *Implication:* Cost analysis can inform healthcare policy and resource allocation, ensuring cost-effective patient care.

Addressing these research gaps can lead to improved surgical techniques, better patient outcomes, and enhanced safety in laparoscopic myomectomy. More comprehensive and high-quality studies are needed to fill these gaps and guide clinical practice.

8.6 ROBOTIC MYOMECTOMY

Rooma Sinha, Amrutha Pentakota

Q1. What are the specific indications when you would prefer robotic myomectomy compared to traditional laparoscopic myomectomy?

Draft recommendations:

a. *Age:* Young women seeking pregnancy where precise enucleation of fibroid and a subsequent robust repair is important for future child-bearing. On the other side of the spectrum, older women with multiple co morbidities where a prolonged general anesthesia is a concern are benefited with robotic myomectomy. With an experienced surgeon and team, the time for robotic myomectomy is often less than laparoscopic myomectomy.
b. *Unmarried:* As conversion rates to laparotomy are reported less when compared to laparoscopic myomectomy. Due to enhanced visual aids, fiber to fiber dissection is possible helping in preserving the healthy uterine tissues to the maximum.
c. *Obese patients:* Robotic surgery is recommended in patients with high BMI. The long length of the instruments and ports being held by the robotic arms helps the surgeon to operate on obese patients with ease.

d. *Pain sensitive:* Post-operative pain is less with robotic surgery. This can be attributed to the fact that the manipulative movement is more at the distal wristed end and not at the abdominal wall level.
e. *Oddly located and multiple myomas:* Inaccessible locations of the fibroid on laparoscopy like the deeply seated cervical fibroids, endo-wrist movements of the robot play a pivotal role allowing easy access for precise dissection. The robotic endo wrist provides 7 degrees of freedom which enables easy access.
f. *Ease of suturing:* The endo-wristed movement of the robotic instruments allows good rangc of dexterity and suturing can be accomplished mimicking the open surgery movements.
g. *Early resumption to work:* Mostly performed as a day care procedure. Patients experience the leverage of early resumption to work due to the assuring post-operative comfort level.
h. In conclusion, robotics is an advanced laparoscopic procedure with all the benefits a conventional laparoscopy.

Summary of evidence: In a study by *Mothes et al., 2023*, authors have encountered no difference between young and old population when robotic surgery was taken into consideration, nevertheless, it did not carry a statistical significance. A meta-analysis by *Wang et al., 2018*, concluded through their study that robotic myomectomy has lesser conversion rate when compared to laparoscopic and open. *Nobbenhuis et al., BJOG, 2022* in sync with the finding concluded that Robotic surgeries have a less conversion rate when compared to conventional laparoscopy. If not directly pertaining to myomectomy alone, studies have shown that usage of a robot has benefits when compared to conventional laparoscopy with heavy as well as obese BMI (as per WHO classification) *Nobbenhuis et al., BJOG, 2022*. This is confirmed in the study by *Sinha et al. in Journal of Robotic Surgery, 2023. Leaf et al., JMIG, 2024* in their study found that with trained professionals performing the minimal invasive surgery with cell salvage technique, the rate of allogenic blood transfusion risk is as less as 1%. From the authors experience, in a study of 177 patients, 116 underwent Robotic myomectomy (RM) while 61 patients underwent Laparoscopic Myomectomy (LM). It was found that RM group had significantly less blood loss (115.43 ± 79.43 vs. 340.98 ± 453.9 mL, $p \leq 0.0001$), even in the absence of any cell salvage techniques. To substantiate this, *Parades et al., GMIT, 2024,* performed a systematic review on “Myomectomy: Choosing the Surgical Approach” and found out that finer dissection, suturing of tissues with poor access is better with robotic surgery than that with abdominal or laparoscopic myomectomies. *Wong et al.* described a study by *Hannah et al.* which stated that with gaze down vision, the execution time and performance are enhanced. In sync with these observations, *Leaf et al., JMIG, 2024* in their 4year retrospective study with the aim of studying the "Feasibility and Perioperative Outcomes of Minimally Invasive Higher Order Myomectomy" have studied 735 women undergoing laparoscopic/robotic myomectomies concluded that patients with higher order myomas (>10 in number) are more benefited with minimal invasive techniques with less conversion to laparotomy. To substantiate, *Mourad et al., meta-analysis, 2024, JORS* through their study, found that patients who underwent open myomectomy stayed for significantly longer time than those in the robotic group. Cumulative analytical data of ten studies represents a mean difference of –1.57 days (–2.0, –1.14), in appreciation of robotics. In a meta-analysis of 20 studies by *Wang et al., 2018,* concluded that the number of complications (OR 0.56, $p=0.03$), length of hospital stay (WMD –1.74, $p<0.00001$) is significantly less with robotic myomectomies.

Q2. What are the criteria for selecting patients who are ideal candidates for robotic myomectomy?

Draft recommendations:

a. Anticipated intra-operative surgical challenges due to previous myomectomy or other multiple surgeries. History of previous complicated surgical sequelae ending in re-exploration.
b. Associated endometriosis or adenomyosis.
c. In frozen pelvis surgeries where tracing the ureter or bladder delineation is of pivotal importance is an ideal candidate. An in-built firefly technology can guide the operating surgeon navigate with ease using the visual clue.

Summary of evidence: *Nobbenhuis et al., BJOG, 2022* have stated, in the absence of a standardization to grade complexity of a surgery, it is perplexing to categorize as to which is a complex surgery and which isn't one. In this process, authors have included various conditions like previous abdominal surgeries, pelvic and pelvic floor surgeries, extensive recto vaginal endometriosis, large retro peritoneal masses, higher BMIs as a few complex surgeries. Authors stated that and Robotic Assisted Laparoscopy is well established for its performance in benign gynecological conditions especially in tubal surgeries and myomectomies. However, authors also have mentioned the limitations in the existing data to have a better evidence based opinion. *Guan X et al., 2016* presented the benefits of using the in-built firefly technology of daVinci for picking up endometriotic lesions and their dissection.

Q3. What are the benefits of robotic assistance in myomectomy?

Draft recommendations:

a. Blood loss is minimal due to the precise dissection into the appropriate planes along with enhanced visualization.

b. Operating time is relatively less. With better vision and approachable endo-wristed arms, often the difficulty of the surgery is minimized contributing to the less surgical time.
c. Stereoscopic vision provides depth perception, and the digital zoom feature of robot makes better visualization of pathology. Conventional 2D laparoscopic surgery doesn't provide the depth perception and results in visual as well as mental fatigue to the surgeon.
d. The dexterity of robotic instruments is wide and apt for dissection. The surgeon can have an autonomous control over the camera and all the working arms giving her/him a near control of surgical field.
e. The stereoscopic immersive vision of the surgeon's console mimics the open surgery with an illusion of sitting over the patient in the midline is a major boon robot offers which a 3-D laparoscopy cannot provide. The ipsilateral and contralateral surgical difficulties of laparoscopy are waved off in robotics due to head on vision of the operative field.
f. A rare human error of touching the surrounding structures/ major vessels with the risky electrosurgical equipment is nullified completely due to stable tremor free robotic arms.
g. Even in extremely lean patients, the robotic platform can be used with ease.
h. The robotic arms can maneuver in tight spaces and around complex anatomical structures effortlessly. In rare cases of parasitic fibroids/ uterine myomas in deep in pouch or near the anterior and lateral pelvic wall laparoscopic dissection is challenging which can be easily overcome using a robot
i. Even obese patients with high BMIs can be operated upon comfortably due to the long length of the robotic instruments with an added benefit of easy maneuverability.
j. Ergonomics of the surgeon is well addressed in robotics giving the operating surgeon a comfortable position to work for longer hours effortlessly.

Summary of evidence: In a meta-analysis by *Wang et al., 2018*, a comparison between abdominal, laparoscopic and robotic procedures of estimated blood loss (WMD –77.74, $p<0.00001$), and numbers of transfusions (OR 0.25, $p<0.0001$) showed the exceptional results in favor of robotic myomectomy with high statistical significance. *Applebaum et al., 2024, JMIG,* have noted that chances of Blood transfusion with OM group is 6 times higher that of MIM group (2.8% v/s 13.0%; $p<.001$). However, the evidence available is not in sync with author's findings. In a latest article by *Applebaum et al., 2024, JMIG,* 27,728 (MIM - 39.9%; OM - 60.1%) patients were studied and noted that Mean operative times (SD) were 164.6 (82.0) minutes for MIM and 129.2 (67.0) minutes for OM MIM (39.9%). It is imperative to understand that in the background of already existing laparoscopic skills by multiple personnel, and with surgeons slowly evolving into robotics in the recent times, more literature is required in the field of robotics for a better comparison of operative time. In a study by Wong et al., the authors have described the visual advantages the robotic console provided. In a *meta-analysis by Mourad et al., 2024,* authors have concluded that robotic surgery has revolutionized the approach to myomectomy in terms of better dexterity, lesser blood loss and improved overall outcomes. In a recently published systematic review by *Parades et al., GMIT, 2024,* found that dexterity, along with the increased degree of freedom in association with eminent 3-D visualization, the hand eye co-ordination is paramount. *Sinha et al., 2021,* in a study published on robotic surgery in 111 pediatric age group children concluded to have successful results using the same adult console. *Nobbenhuis et al., BJOG, 2022,* authors have described that in obese patients with BMI >30kg/sq. m and those with lung issues, a robotic surgery can offer the best compared to other modalities. In addition, authors also stated that Work related musculoskeletal problems are known to depreciate the productivity and longevity of surgeons which is in sync with our recommendation.

Q4. What are the limitations of robotic modality when it comes to myomectomy?

Draft recommendations:

a. Requires a bigger operating room to accommodate all the three parts of the robotic platform.
b. The assistant surgeons and the nurses need a specialized training in robotics to understand the equipment and its usage.
c. Tactile feedback is a lacking feature which can lead to suture breakage. However, it can be overcome with stereoscopic 3D-vision provided by the robotic platform which is also called as "Visual haptics".
d. The capital cost of acquiring the Robotic equipment at present is expensive. Cost can be brought down by increased volume of cases.

Summary of evidence: *Wong SW et al., 2023* support our draft recommendations of improved stereopsis with robotic console. *Wu CZ, 2019* in their review of cost effectiveness with robotic surgeries concluded that with increasing surgeons experience and by decreasing the post operative complications to a bare minimal the equipment charges are soon going to lower down making it accessible option for everyone.

Q5. In what situations would you prefer traditional laparoscopy over robotic myomectomy?

Draft recommendations: Robotic surgery is advanced version of conventional laparoscopy. All cases with large, oddly located, multiple fibroids will benefit with the robotic platform as the wrist like maneuverability makes it easier not only to enucleate these fibroids but also to suture effectively in odd angles. Hence all cases that can be operated using conventional laparoscopy can be operated using the robotic approach.

Summary of evidence: *Gkegkes et al., 2020,* through their review article concluded in sync with the draft recommendation that robotic myomectomies are of better benefit over conventional laparoscopy or open surgeries. *Sheng Y et al., 2023* with their metanalysis have stated that robotic myomectomy is superior to laparoscopic myomectomy in multiple aspects namely intraoperative bleeding, less blood transfusion rates, post operative hospital stay and post operative complications except for operative time. *However, in the situation where laparoscopy is well established with existing "trained" status, it is imperative to note that robotics is newly evolving technique and it would be a biased result when operative time is being compared at this level.*

Q6. What are the potential complications associated with robotic myomectomy, and how can they be managed intraoperatively and postoperatively?

Draft recommendations:

a. Complications with robotic myomectomy are similar to laparoscopic myomectomy as both are minimally invasive procedure.
b. Conversion rates are lesser with robotic approach when compared to laparoscopic surgery.

Summary of evidence: In a meta-analysis of 20 studies by *Wang et al., 2018,* concluded that the number of complications (OR 0.56, $p=0.03$), length of hospital stay (WMD −1.74, $p<0.00001$) is significantly less with robotic myomectomies

Q7. How do you compare the recovery time and postoperative outcomes between patients undergoing robotic myomectomy and those undergoing traditional laparoscopic and open myomectomy?

Draft recommendations:

a. Robotic Myomectomy can be done as a day care procedure. Post-operative complications are less compared to the open myomectomies.
b. The reported re-admission rates are less with robotic surgeries.

Summary of evidence: In a meta-analysis by *Wang et al., 2018,* concluded that the number of complications (OR 0.56, $p=0.03$), length of hospital stay (WMD −1.74, $p<0.00001$) is significantly less with robotic myomectomies. In a latest article by *Applebaum et al., 2024, JMIG,* 27,728 were studied and a significant difference of values in post-operative complications between MIM (Minimal Invasive Myomectomy) and OM (Open myomectomy) groups were noted. Composite complications: MIM v/s OM (5.5% v/s 15.8%; p <.001); Minor complications MIM v/s OM (4.7% v/s14.8%; p <.001); Major complications MIM v/s OM (1.0% v/s 1.9%; p <.001). Looking into the readmission rates, comparing MIM v/s OM (1.4% 1.9%; p <.001) though the values are seemingly similar in both the groups, it is noteworthy that lower readmission rate associated with MIM was statistically significant. Authors also added that Re-operative procedure rate was double with OM when compared to MIM. (1.0% v/s 0.5%; p <.001)

Q8. What are the challenges one can encounter in robotic myomectomy and how can one solve them?

Draft recommendations: At present there are two challenges with robotic surgery.

- Lack of haptic—This can cause suture breakage in the learning curve. With experience and the use of "visual haptics" this can be overcome.
- Increased cost—with increased volume and multi-specialty involvement the institutions can reduce cost. With more and more types of platform now available, the cost is expected to recued over the coming years.

Summary of evidence: *Wong et al.*, in sync have stated "The daVinci console returns the screen in line with the surgeon hands" is a visual feedback which replicates a live surgery. The initial expenditure to acquire the robotic equipment is high. But with increased usage for wide variety of cases by multiple surgeons, the costs can be brought down soon. *Wu CZ et al.* in their review article on strategies to improve cost effectiveness with robotics concluded that less conversion rates and decreased hospital stay, greatly contribute to overall cost reduction associated with a surgery.

8.7 WHAT IS THE CURRENT ROLE OF VAGINAL MYOMECTOMY AND vNOTES MYOMECTOMY?

Suyash Naval

Draft recommendations:

- *The specific role of vaginal myomectomy in comparison to laparotomy, laparoscopy, and hysteroscopy cannot be accurately determined and is not thoroughly evaluated in the existing research.*
- *It is advisable to limit vaginal myomectomy to easily reachable posterior myomas, without considering its application in other cases.*
- *vNOTES is equally safe and effective in uterine myomectomy compared with multiport and single-port laparoscopy, and can be used as a routine procedure only for carefully selected patients.*

- *vNOTES patients recover faster after surgery, but still attention should be paid to preoperative evaluation, strengthen preoperative disinfection and vaginal preparation and timely conversion during surgery.*
- *vNOTES myomectomy should be performed by doctors trained and experienced in this technique, and routine use of antibiotics to prevent postoperative infection is suggested.*
- *Large fundal myomas, multiple myomas, cervical myomas and large broad ligament myomas can be considered as relative contraindications for vNOTES approach.*
- *The current evidence is classified as level III, a well-planned cohort or randomized research is recommended to evaluate the role of vaginal myomectomy and vNOTES myomectomy.*

DISCUSSION AND REVIEW OF LITERATURE

There is limited information available in scientific literature regarding the number of patients who have undergone vaginal myomectomy. The research conducted on this topic are generally categorized as level III evidence. Consequently, it is not feasible to draw definitive conclusions on this technique. Nevertheless, the current practicality of this myomectomy procedure appears to be satisfactory.

The procedure carries a variable probability of conversion to laparotomy, as reported in different studies. The assessment of risk factors for conversion to laparotomy is lacking. However, according to several authors, the placement of the myoma in the fundus and the presence of substantial volumes of myoma are considered to be risk factors. According to certain authors, based on their expertise, it is recommended to employ this technique just for cases when there is a solitary posterior myoma of restricted dimensions (<8 cm) that can be detected during vaginal examination.

The literature does not provide sufficient data to accurately determine the frequency of perioperative and postoperative problems. Nevertheless, these rates do not appear to be higher when compared to procedures conducted using laparotomy, laparoscopy, or hysteroscopy, which also carry the risk of synechiae. Possible causes of postoperative fever include hematoma or the presence of a vaginal drain. Several publications posit that there is a potential for heightened risk of postoperative pelvic infection following vaginal myomectomy.

The clear assessment of the specific role of vaginal myomectomy in comparison to laparotomy, laparoscopy, and hysteroscopy is lacking in the literature. The literature either lacks reports or studies on the advantages of one technique over another in terms of procedure duration, hospital stay length, and cost. Nevertheless, it is advisable to limit vaginal myomectomy to posterior myomas that may be easily reached, and laparoscopy should not be used to assess its feasibility. Although the data is classified as level III, a well-planned cohort or randomized research could still be valuable.

New micro-invasive gynecological technology called vNOTES (vaginal natural orifice transluminal endoscopic surgery) is being employed worldwide. For ovarian cystectomy, salpingectomy, myomectomy, hysterectomy, and early-stage cancer surgery, it is less invasive. vNOTES lowers pain, speeds recovery, and cosmetically covers surgical incisions.

Some studies have explored vNOTES myomectomy potential. Qiannan Hou et al. (2022), compared three minimally invasive fibroid removal procedures: multiport laparoscopy, Single port laparoscopy and vNOTES. Patients in each group had similar backgrounds, establishing demographic baseline homogeneity. It has been demonstrated that vNOTES surgery did not affect subsequent pregnancy and delivery, although further evidence is needed.

Operative time varied greatly between the three groups. Port number significantly affected surgical time, except for fibroids and pelvic adhesion. Umbilicus or vaginal single-port surgery takes longer than multiport laparoscopy. Under the same conditions, single-port laparoscopic surgery took 25 minutes longer. Single-port laparoscopy's issues—instrument interference, no aid, passive surgeon position—are the main cause. The time extension is moderate and small. Robotic surgery improved these concerns with tool articulation and precision. Safe and effective single-port specimen removal prevents morcellation-induced tumor spread. VNOTES remove specimens better than navels because the vaginal wall is more elastic and less muscle relaxant-dependent. The number of uterine fibroids and operation time caused intraoperative bleeding differences between the three groups, not the surgical approach. Five patients with intraoperative blood loss >500 mL was eliminated from statistical analysis due to considerable dispersion. Each of these five patients was investigated separately. Three were in vNOTES, two in LESS. There was no specific cause of intraoperative bleeding, however all uterine fibroids were larger than 8 cm, including one 15 cm. The multiport group lost less blood than LESS when the fibroid diameter was large. The surgery went well without transfer despite considerable bleeding.

Comparing postoperative recovery time with the three groups, vNOTES proved superior. Thus, postoperative hospitalization was cheaper and shorter. Here are the main causes of early postoperative recovery. Initially, vNOTES surgery is done in the pelvis with little upper abdominal impact. Second, the intestine was transferred to the pelvis before surgery to avoid instruments touching the intestinal canal. It would reduce intestinal stimulation. The surgical viewpoint is upward, so blood collects between the endoscopic body and the target place, therefore blood should be cleaned constantly for clear eyesight. Postoperative residual blood volume in the abdominal cavity is considerably reduced, reducing chemical stimulation, inflammatory factor release, and intestinal function recovery. Finally, visceral nerves rule the posterior vaginal fornix, where vNOTES entry is created. Unlike the abdominal approach that irritates or damages somatosensory nerves. Since vNOTES patients have less postoperative pain, they can stand faster and promote intestinal peristalsis.

Despite these benefits, a greater infection risk was observed after vNOTES by Qiannan Hou et al. (2022), contradicting previous studies. Note that not all myomectomies use vNOTES. With its narrow field of view and surgical instrument scope, vNOTES cannot treat fibroids at the bottom of the uterus or broad ligament. Myomectomy using vNOTES is not performed for multiple uterine fibroids in the anterior and posterior walls of the uterus because it requires two vault openings, which causes greater trauma and manipulation. This technique involves fibroids at the site and should not be performed on patients with severe endometriosis, pelvic infection, and uncured vaginitis. Pelvic surgery and obesity are safe.

8.8 ROLE OF HYSTERECTOMY FOR FIBROIDS

Sunita Tandulwadkar, Rashmika Gandhi, Vatsla Vats

Q1. Indications for hysterectomy in fibroid uterus.

Draft recommendations:

1. Hysterectomy is recommended for women with large symptomatic fibroids who do not desire future fertility, after comprehensive counseling about the long-term risks.
2. It should be considered for symptomatic women seeking definitive treatment after other conservative or medical treatment modalities have failed.

Discussion:

- Hysterectomy serves as a definitive surgical management option for Abnormal Uterine Bleeding associated with leiomyomas (AUB-L) and bulk symptoms (pain, pressure symptoms, constipation) in patients who do not desire future childbearing. This recommendation is contingent upon thorough counseling and education about the procedure.
- While the management of uterine fibroids depends on various factors—including the size and location of fibroids, the patient's age, and desire to preserve fertility—the decision should be individualized based on access to therapy and surgeon expertise, risk of complications, and need for subsequent surgical interventions.
- Hysterectomy should only be considered when other treatments have failed, are contraindicated, or declined, and the woman no longer wishes to retain her uterus and fertility.

- Expectant management may be appropriate for asymptomatic uterine fibroids. Studies show significant improvement in hemoglobin levels and quality of life post-hysterectomy. However, the procedure is associated with long-term morbidity such as loss of fertility and potential increase in cardiovascular and cognitive risks, especially when performed with bilateral oophorectomy, which is rarely indicated for fibroids alone.

Research gap: Current guidelines do not provide clear size or age thresholds for recommending hysterectomy in the management of fibroids, which may lead to variability in clinical practice. More research is needed to define the specific fibroid dimensions and patient age factors that would most benefit from hysterectomy versus conservative management. This gap highlights the necessity for developing precise, evidence-based criteria to guide clinical decisions effectively.

Q2. What are the factors determining approach and route of hysterectomy?

Draft recommendations:

1. The most minimally invasive route (vaginal hysterectomy) should be preferred whenever feasible for benign conditions.
2. Laparoscopic hysterectomy is recommended as a preferable alternative to abdominal hysterectomy when vaginal hysterectomy is not possible or indicated.

Discussion:

- The choice of approach for hysterectomy has evolved to include multiple methods beyond traditional abdominal hysterectomy, each with its specific advantages and constraints. Surgical routes can vary from vaginal, abdominal, to laparoscopic, including newer methods like robotics and vNOTES.
- The choice of hysterectomy route for benign causes should be determined by factors such as the size and shape of the uterus, accessibility and mobility of the uterus, extent of extrauterine disease, the need for concurrent procedures, surgeon training and experience, available hospital technology and support, whether the case is emergent or elective, and patient preferences after informed consent.
- Systematic reviews and meta-analyses suggest that minimally invasive approaches (vaginal, laparoscopic) should be the first choice for benign conditions due to their documented advantages over abdominal hysterectomy. For instance, vaginal hysterectomy is associated with shorter operation times, decreased blood loss, shorter hospital stays, and fewer complications compared to laparoscopic hysterectomy. However, it may be limited by the size of the fibroid uterus and the patient's anatomy. On the other hand, laparoscopic hysterectomy shows improved outcomes

like faster return to normal activities and reduced risks of surgical site infection, though it carries a higher risk of urinary tract injuries and requires more extended operation times compared to abdominal methods.

Research gap: While the advantages of minimally invasive techniques are well documented, there is a lack of comprehensive guidelines that specify which patient characteristics or uterine sizes best suit each surgical route. Further studies are needed to establish clear, evidence-based criteria that can help surgeons choose the most appropriate technique based on individual patient cases.

Q3. What are the merits of robot assisted hysterectomy for fibroid uterus?

Draft recommendations: The role of robotic assistance in executing laparoscopic hysterectomy for fibroid uterus remains uncertain.

Discussion:

- Robot-assisted laparoscopic hysterectomy, a variation on traditional laparoscopic techniques, has been employed to a limited extent for hysterectomy procedures. It has not demonstrated superior surgical outcomes compared to traditional laparoscopy.
- The potential benefits of robot-assisted laparoscopy include enhanced visualization through three-dimensional imaging, superior mechanical capabilities, improved ergonomics, and a potentially quicker learning curve for many surgeons. These advantages may be particularly beneficial in avoiding open abdominal hysterectomy, especially for patients who are severely obese or have extensive pelvic adhesions. Nonetheless, specific patient subgroups that would benefit most from robot-assisted hysterectomy remain unclear.
- Studies comparing robot-assisted to traditional laparoscopic hysterectomy have shown that while the robotic approach can increase operating times, it does not significantly alter hospital stay lengths. Cost, training, and accessibility also remain significant barriers to the widespread adoption of robotic-assisted hysterectomy.

Q4. What structured counseling and informed consent must be undertaken for hysterectomy as well as the route of surgery?

Draft recommendations:

- The informed consent process must provide patients with essential information to aid decision-making.
- A detailed consent form, written in the patient's understandable language, should include patient details, procedure name, route/approach of hysterectomy, benefits, risks, and complications involved, alternative procedures available, consent for anesthesia and blood transfusion,

patient's authorization and declaration, surgeon's details, and signatures of the patient and/or witness with the date and time of consent.

Discussion:

- Structured counseling and obtaining informed consent are pivotal in preparing patients for surgery. This process ensures that patients are fully informed of the benefits and risks associated with the surgery, respects their autonomy, and builds trust between the patient and the healthcare provider. Effective consent encompasses several key elements:
  - *Competence/Capacity:* Assessing the patient's ability to understand the information provided and make a decision.
  - *Disclosure:* Providing comprehensive information about the procedure's intended benefits and potential risks.
  - *Understanding:* Ensuring that the patient understands the information provided.
  - *Voluntariness:* Confirming that the decision is made without coercion.
- For hysterectomy, a shared decision-making approach is crucial. This should include a thorough discussion with the patient about the specific technique and route of the surgery, considering the individual's priorities and medical context. The consent form should comprehensively cover all potential outcomes and alternative treatments available.

Research gap: Research should focus on developing innovative approaches to improve patient comprehension and satisfaction with the consent process, especially in diverse populations with varying levels of health literacy.

Q5. What is the role of ovarian conservation during hysterectomy for fibroids?

Draft recommendations:

- The decision regarding ovarian conservation or removal during hysterectomy for benign indications like fibroids should be individualized.
- For premenopausal patients undergoing hysterectomy for benign indications, ovarian conservation is generally recommended to preserve ovarian function and mitigate the long-term health risks associated with premature menopause.
- Elective oophorectomy should only be considered for patients with specific risk factors or those prioritizing ovarian cancer prevention over potential long-term health consequences.

Discussion:

- The decision to perform oophorectomy at the time of hysterectomy for benign conditions such as fibroids balances the risks and benefits of ovarian conservation versus removal. Traditionally, bilateral salpingo-oophorectomy (BSO) was frequently recommended to premenopausal women to reduce ovarian cancer risk and avoid future surgeries related to ovarian pathology. However, recent insights into the long-term health effects of oophorectomy have prompted a shift toward ovarian conservation, particularly among younger patients.

- Ovarian conservation helps preserve hormonal function, which can reduce risks such as cardiovascular disease and osteoporosis linked to premature menopause. Current data suggest that oophorectomy before natural menopause may increase all-cause mortality, cardiovascular disease, and cognitive decline risks. Moreover, studies indicate that ovarian conservation does not significantly elevate ovarian cancer risk in average-risk women and might protect against other malignancies like breast cancer.
- Conversely, elective oophorectomy might be considered for patients nearing or past menopausal age who have a high ovarian cancer risk or prioritize cancer prevention over the potential risks of long-term health issues. This decision must be carefully weighed against the evidence of increased risks of chronic diseases and decreased quality of life associated with surgical menopause.

Research gap: There is a need for further research to definitively quantify the benefits and risks associated with ovarian conservation versus removal in various patient subgroups, particularly to refine guidelines for premenopausal women with different risk profiles.

Q6: What is the role of uterine artery ligation in certain cases of hysterectomy?

Draft recommendations: Uterine artery ligation is recommended in certain cases of hysterectomy, particularly for large fibroids, severe endometriosis, adenomyosis or prior pelvic surgeries, to reduce intraoperative blood loss, facilitate tissue dissection, and improve surgical outcomes.

Discussion:

- Uterine artery ligation is a critical step in certain complex hysterectomies. It is particularly advantageous in cases with distorted pelvic anatomy caused by large fibroids, endometriosis, or prior pelvic surgeries. Early ligation of the uterine arteries significantly reduces intraoperative blood loss, enhancing visibility and simplifying subsequent surgical steps.
- In cases of suspected malignancy, uterine artery ligation can aid in achieving hemostasis, which is crucial for optimal surgical resection and minimizing complications. Studies also indicate that prophylactic uterine artery ligation may facilitate tissue dissection in cases of severe endometriosis or adenomyosis, reducing the risk of damage to adjacent structures.

- While generally safe, uterine artery ligation requires careful surgical technique to avoid complications like ureteric injury. It is a versatile step that can be tailored to individual surgical needs, depending on uterine size, pathology, and the patient's overall condition.

Research gap: While the benefits of uterine artery ligation are well-documented, there is a lack of high-quality evidence specifically comparing outcomes in patients who undergo uterine artery ligation versus those who do not in similar surgical scenarios. Further research is needed to:

- Quantify the reduction in blood loss and operative time in specific patient subgroups.
- Evaluate the long-term outcomes and complications associated with uterine artery ligation in complex hysterectomies.

Develop evidence-based criteria for selecting patients who would benefit most from this technique.

Q7. What is the ideal follow-up care following hysterectomy?

Draft recommendations:

- Patients should receive standard postoperative care including pain management, wound care, and monitoring for any signs of infection or complications. Early ambulation should be encouraged to reduce the risk of thromboembolic events.
- Schedule the first follow-up visit within 4-6 weeks post-surgery to assess the healing of the surgical site, evaluate for any immediate postoperative complications, and discuss any concerns the patient might have regarding recovery.
- Annual examinations should be recommended to monitor for any long-term complications or new symptoms that could indicate issues such as vault prolapse or adhesions.

Discussion:

- The ideal follow-up care for hysterectomy patients should encompass both immediate and long-term health needs. Immediate postoperative care focuses on recovery from surgery, managing pain, and preventing complications.
- Special attention might be necessary for psychological support, as some patients may experience emotional distress or feelings of loss post-hysterectomy.
- Additionally, lifestyle adjustments and hormone replacement therapy (if applicable) should be discussed to manage symptoms of menopause and reduce long-term health risks.

Research gap: Current guidelines on the optimal duration and frequency of follow-up post-hysterectomy are based on general recommendations.

Specific evidence-based guidelines tailored to different types of hysterectomy and patient demographic profiles are needed to optimize long-term outcomes and patient satisfaction.

Q8. Should unplanned hysterectomy be offered based on intraoperative findings suspicious of sarcoma?

Draft recommendations: If suspicious findings of sarcoma are identified during a procedure intended for benign conditions, the decision to convert to hysterectomy should be approached with caution. Intraoperative frozen section analysis may be utilized to guide decision making if available.

Discussion:

- Unplanned hysterectomy during surgery initially intended for benign conditions can be a challenging decision, particularly if sarcoma is suspected. The risks of spreading malignant cells should be balanced against the immediate benefits of tumor removal.
- Collaborative decision-making with oncologists and pathologists during surgery is critical to optimize patient outcomes and adhere to oncological safety standards. Engage a multidisciplinary team including gynecologic oncologists when possible before proceeding with an unplanned hysterectomy.
- Ensure that preoperative consent includes discussion about the potential for unexpected findings and the possibility of extended surgery, such as hysterectomy, to allow for informed decision-making in real time.

Research gap: There is a need for more robust data and established protocols to guide surgeons on the management of unexpected findings suggestive of sarcoma during pelvic surgeries. Further research should focus on the outcomes of immediate versus delayed hysterectomy after the discovery of potential malignancies.

BIBLIOGRAPHY

1. ACOG Committee on Practice Bulletins–Gynecology. Practice Bulletin No. 183: Management of symptomatic uterine fibroids. Obstet Gynecol. 2017;130(5)
2. ACOG Committee Opinion. The use of morcellation in gynecologic surgery. Obstet Gynecol. 2018;131(4).
3. Advincula AP, Xu X. Laparoscopic myomectomy: a comparison of various techniques. J Gynecol Surg. 2004;20(3):99-108.
4. Agostini A, Gerbeau S, Al Nakid M, et al. Complications of vaginal myomectomy by posterior colpotomy. Eur J Obstet Gynaecol Reprod Biol. 2008;138:100-4.
5. Albright BB, Witte T, Tofte AN, et al. Robotic versus laparoscopic hysterectomy for benign disease: a systematic review and meta-analysis of randomized trials. J Minimally Invasive Gynecol. 2016;23:18-27.
6. American College of Surgeons: Surgical guidelines for the management of unexpected gynecologic malignancy. Ann Surg Oncol. 2019;26(7):2023-31.

7. Applebaum J, Kim EK, Ewy J, et al. Operative Time and Accrual of Postoperative Complications in Minimally Invasive Versus Open Myomectomy. J Minim Invasive Gynecol. 2024:S1553-4650(24)00213-9.
8. Badiglian-Filho L, Fukazawa EM, Faloppa C, Baiocchi G. Ovarian sparing cystectomy for borderline serous tumor through vNOTES (vaginal Natural Orifices Transluminal Endoscopic Surgery). Int J Gynecol Cancer. 2020;30(8):1253-4.
9. Badiglian-Filho L, Fukazawa EM, Faloppa CC, et al. VNOTES (Vaginal Natural Orifices Transluminal Endoscopic Surgery) myomectomy through anterior cul-de-sac approach on the bicornuate uterus. J Gynecol Obstet Hum Reprod. 2021;50(1):101911.
10. Baekelandt J, Noori N, Hofmann L, et al. Standardised step by step approach to adnexectomy by Vaginal Natural Orifice Transluminal Endoscopic Surgery. Eur J Obstet Gynecol Reprod Biol. 2022;274:160-5.
11. Baekelandt JF, De Mulder PA, Le Roy I, et al. Transvaginal natural orifice transluminal endoscopic surgery (vNOTES) adnexectomy for benign pathology compared with laparoscopic excision (NOTABLE): a protocol for a randomised controlled trial. BMJ Open. 2018;8(1):e018059.
12. Bedaiwy MA. Uterine artery occlusion at myomectomy? Toward a better definition of the indications. Fertil Steril. 2019;111(4):685-6.
13. Bennett GL. Uterine rupture after myomectomy: A review of the literature. Obstet Gynecol. 2021;137(4):755-61.
14. Berek JS, Chalas E, Edelson M, et al. Prophylactic and risk-reducing bilateral salpingo-oophorectomy: recommendations based on risk of ovarian cancer. Obstetr Gynecol. 20210;116:733.
15. Bettocchi S, Sardo AD, Ceci O, et al. A new hysteroscopic technique for the preparation of partially intramural myomas in office setting (OPPIuM technique): a pilot study. J Minim Invasive Gynecol. 2009;16(6):748-54.
16. Buhur A, Necdet O. Comparison of laparoscopic and open myomectomy in a tertiary hospital: a retrospective cohort study. Comprehens Med. 2024;16(2): 112-7.
17. Burgess L. Safety measures in laparoscopic morcellation: a systematic review. Surg Endosc. 2017;31(5):2077-86.
18. Capmas P, Levaillant JM, Fernandez H. Surgical techniques and outcome in the management of submucous fibroids. Curr Opin Obstet Gynecol. 2013;25:332-8.
19. Capozzi VA, Armano G, Rosati A, et al. The robotic single-port platform for gynecologic surgery: a systematic review of the literature and meta-analysis. Updates Surg. 2021;73(3):1155-67.
20. Casini ML, Rossi F, Agostini R, et al. Effects of the position of fibroids on fertility. Gynecol Endocrinol. 2006;22:106-9.
21. Chang KM, Chen MJ, Lee MH, et al. Fertility and pregnancy outcomes after uterine artery occlusion with or without myomectomy. Taiwanese J Obstetr Gynecol. 2012;51(3):331-5.
22. Clark NA, Mumford SL, Segars JH. Reproductive Impact of MRI guided focused ultrasound surgery for fibroids: a systematic review of the evidence. Curr Opin Obstet Gynecol. 2014;26:151-61.
23. Clement R. Surgical approaches for the removal of large fibroids: a comparative study. Int J Gynaecol Obstet. 2020;148(3):306-11.

24. Cohen SL, Einarsson JI, Wang KC, et al. Contained power morcellation within an insufflated isolation bag. Obstetr Gynecol. 2016;128(3):481-5.
25. Cohen SL. Manual morcellation versus power morcellation in laparoscopic myomectomy: a comparative study. J Minim Invasive Gynecol. 2014;21(5):854-8.
26. Committee Opinion No. 701: Choosing the Route of Hysterectomy for Benign Disease. Obstet Gynecol. 2017;129(6):e155-9.
27. Cucinella G, Granese R, Calagna G, et al. Parasitic myomas after laparoscopic surgery: an emerging complication in the use of morcellator? Fertil Steril. 2011; 96(2):e90-6.
28. Davies A, Hart R, Magos AL. The excision of uterine myomas by vaginal myomectomy: a retrospective study. Fertil Steril. 1999;71:961-4.
29. De La Cruz MSD, Buchanan EM. (2017) 'Uterine fibroids: diagnosis and treatment', Am Fam Phys. 2017;95(2):100-7.
30. De Vries BR. Long-term health surveillance after hysterectomy: European consensus recommendations. Euro J Obstetr Gynecol Reprod Biol. 2022;267: 134-43.
31. Deng Y. Containment systems in laparoscopic myomectomy: enhancing patient safety. Surg Endosc. 2017;31(4):1520-5.
32. Desai P, Pisat S, Desai S. The "Trick" Knot—A Modified Technique of the Removable "Shoelace" Knot for Temporary Ligation of the Uterine Artery at Its Origin. Journal of Minim Invas Gynecol. 2022;29(12):1291.
33. Desai VB. Minimally invasive approaches for myomectomy: A review. Curr Opin Obstet Gynecol. 2015;27(4):311-7.
34. Di Spiezio Sardo A, Mazzon I, Bramante S, et al. Hysteroscopic myomectomy: A comprehensive review of surgical techniques. Hum Reprod Update. 2008; 14(2):101-19.
35. Donnez J, Hudecek R, Donnez O, et al. Efficacy and safety of repeated use of ulipristal acetate in uterine fibroids. Fertil Steril. 2015;103(2):519-27.e3.
36. Dubin AK, Wei J, Sullivan S, et al. Minilaparotomy versus Laparoscopic myomectomy after cessation of power morcellation: Rate of wound complications. J Minim Invasive Gynecol. 2017;24:946-53.
37. Dueholm M, Forman A, Ingerslev J. Regression of residual tissue after incomplete resection of submucous myomas. Gyneacol Endosc. 1998;7:309-14.
38. Dueholm M, Lundorf E, Hansen ES, et al. Magnetic resonance imaging and transvaginal ultrasonography for the diagnosis of adenomyosis. Fertil Steril. 201;76(3):588-94.
39. Einarsson JI, Vellinga TT, Twijnstra AR, et al. Bidirectional barbed suture: an evaluation of safety and clinical outcomes. JSLS. 2010;14(3):381-5.
40. Einstein MH, Seidman JD. Tissue retrieval in laparoscopic myomectomy: the implications of morcellation. Obstet Gynecol. 2008;112(2 Pt 1):299-304.
41. Emanuel MK, Wamsteker K, Augustinus AMH, et al. Long-term results of hysteroscopic myomectomy for abnormal uttering bleeding. Obstet Gynecol. 1999;93:743-8.
42. Erickson Z, Rocca WA, Smith CY, et al. Time trends in unilateral and bilateral oophorectomy in a geographically defined American population. Obstetr Gynecol. 2022;139:724.
43. Faivre E, Surroca MM, Deffieux X, et al. Vaginal Myomectomy: Literature Review. J Minim Invas Gynecol. 2010;17(2):154-60.

44. Feng D, He L. Pregnancy and childbirth after transvaginal natural orifice transluminal endoscopic surgery for benign gynecological diseases. Int J Gynaecol Obstet. 2021;155(3):551-2.
45. Fiscella K, Eisinger SH, Meldrum S, et al. Effect of mifepristone for symptomatic leiomyomata on quality of life and uterine size: a randomized controlled trial. Obstet Gynecol. 2006;108(6):1381-7.
46. Franklin L. Management of submucosal myoma not completely resected. JMIG. 2019;26(5):787-8.
47. Gkegkes ID, Iatrakis G, Iavazzo PE, et al. Robotic Management of Fibroids: Discussion of Use, Criteria and Advantages. Acta Medica (Hradec Kralove). 2020;63(2):63-6.
48. Godbole RD. Ventricular Tachycardia Caused by Intramyometrial Infiltration of Vasopressin during Laparoscopic Myomectomy: An Anesthesiologist's Nightmare. J Med Sci. 2019;5(2):57-8.
49. Goldstein SR. Fertility preservation in women undergoing myomectomy. Fertil Steril. 2016;105(1):76-81.
50. Goto A, Takeuchi S, Sugimura K, et al. Usefulness of Gd-DTPA contrast-enhanced dynamic MRI and serum determination of LDH and its isozymes in the differential diagnosis of leiomyosarcoma from degenerated leiomyoma of the uterus. Int J Gynecol Cancer. 2002;12(4):354-61.
51. Greenberg JA, Goldman RH. Barbed suture: A review of the technology and clinical uses in obstetrics and gynecology. Rev Obstet Gynecol. 2013;6(3-4):107-15.
52. Guan X, Nguyen MT, Walsh TM, et al. Robotic Single-Site Endometriosis Resection Using Firefly Technology. J Minim Invasive Gynecol. 2016;23(1): 10-1.
53. Hanna GB, Shimi SM, Cuschieri A. Task performance in endoscopic surgery is influenced by location of the image display. Ann Surg. 1998;227(4):481-4.
54. Hata K, Hata T, Maruyama R, et al. Uterine sarcoma: can it be differentiated from uterine leiomyoma with Doppler ultrasonography? A preliminary report. Ultrasound Obstet Gynecol. 2002;9:101-4.
55. Hiratsuka D, Isono W, Tsuchiya A, et al. The effect of temporary uterine artery ligation on laparoscopic myomectomy to reduce intraoperative blood loss: A retrospective case-control study. Eur J Obstetr Gynecol Reprod Biol. 2022;15:100162.
56. Holub Z. Laparoscopic myomectomy: Indications and limits. Ceska Gynekol. 2007;72:64-8.
57. Huang L, Lin YH, Yang Y, et al. Comparative analysis of vaginal natural orifice transluminal endoscopic surgery versus transumbilical laparoendoscopic single-site surgery in ovarian cystectomy. J Obstet Gynaecol Res. 2021;47(2):757-64.
58. Huber D, Hurni Y. Sentinel node biopsy for endometrial cancer by retroperitoneal transvaginal natural orifice transluminal endoscopic surgery: a preliminary study. Front Surg. 2022;9:907548.
59. Informed Consent and Shared Decision Making in Obstetrics and Gynecology: ACOG Committee Opinion, Number 819. Obstet Gynecol. 2021;137(2):e34-e41.
60. Intrauterine Bigatti Shaver. EndoWorld. Gyn 48 7.0 01/2016.
61. Jain N, Singh S. Cervical Fibroids: Techniques for Myomectomy and Hysterectomy. Fibroid Uterus. Boca Raton, Florida, United States: CRC Press. 2020. pp. 80-9.

62. Jin C, Hu Y, Chen XC, et al. Laparoscopic versus open myomectomy: a meta-analysis of randomized controlled trials. Eur J Obstetr Gynecol Reprod Biol. 2009;145(1):14-21
63. Jin C, Hu Y, Chen XC, et al. Laparoscopic versus open myomectomy: a meta-analysis of randomized controlled trials. Eur J Obstetr Gynecol Reprod Biol. 2009;145(1):14-21
64. Karkia R, Giacchino T, Taylor J, et al. Hysterectomy and adenextomy via transvaginal natural orifice transluminal endoscopic surgery (vNOTES): a UK perspective with a case series of 33 patients. Eur J Obstet Gynecol Reprod Biol. 2019;242:29-32.
65. Khan AT, Shehmar M, Gupta JK. Uterine fibroids: Current perspectives. Int J Womens Health. 2014;6:95-114.
66. Khan M. MRI in the evaluation of uterine fibroids. Radiographics. 2019; 39(6):1711-27.
67. Kongnyuy EJ, Wiysonge CS. Interventions to reduce haemorrhage during myomectomy for fibroids. Cochrane Database Syst Rev. 2014;2014(8):CD005355.
68. Laganà AS, Pacheco LA, Tinelli A, et al. Management of asymptomatic submucous myomas in women of reproductive age: a consensus statement from the global congress on hysteroscopy scientific committee. J Minim Invasive Gynecol. 2019;26:381-3.
69. Lasmar R, Lasmar B. Histeroscopia Técnica & Arte, 1st editon. Brazil: Thieme Revinter: Rio de Janeiro; 2021.
70. Lasmar RB, Barrozo PR. Histeroscopia: Uma abordagem pr_atica. Rio de Janeiro: Medsi; 2002.
71. Lasmar RB, Barrozo PRM, Dias R, et al. Submucous myomas: a new presurgical classification to evaluate the viability of hysteroscopic surgical treatment—Preliminary report. JMIG. 2005;12:308-11.
72. Lasmar RB, Lasmar BP, Moawad NS. Hysteroscopic Myomectomy. Medicina (Kaunas). 2022;58(11).
73. Lasmar RB, Lasmar BP. Limiting Factors of Office Hysteroscopic Myomectomy. Hysteroscopy. Berlin/Heidelberg, Germany: Springer; 2017; pp. 357-62.
74. Lawrie TA, Liu H, Lu D, et al. Robot-assisted surgery in gynaecology. Cochrane Database Syst Rev. 2019;4:CD011422.
75. Leaf MC, Lombardo A, Wainger JJ, et al. Feasibility and Perioperative Outcomes of Minimally Invasive Higher Order Myomectomy. J Minim Invasive Gynecol. 2024;31(10):870-4.
76. Lee EJ, Park SJ, Kim Y, et al. Effect and safety of diluted vasopressin injection on bleeding during robot-assisted laparoscopic myomectomy: a protocol for a randomised controlled pilot trial. BMJ Open. 2022;12(9):e056145.
77. Lethaby A, Vollenhoven B, Sowter M. Pre-operative GnRH analogue therapy before hysterectomy or myomectomy for uterine fibroids. Cochrane Database Syst Rev. 2001;(2):CD000547.
78. Lethaby A, Vollenhoven B. Fibroids (uterine myomatosis, leiomyomas). BMJ Clin Evid. 2015;2015:0814.
79. Leung F, Terzibachian JJ, Gay C. The role of frozen section in intraoperative diagnosis of pelvic masses: accuracy and limitations. Gynecol Oncol Rep. 2022;39:100793.

80. Liu J, Lin Q, Blazek K, et al. Transvaginal natural orifice transluminal endoscopic surgery myomectomy: a novel route for uterine myoma removal. J Minim Invasive Gynecol. 2018:25(6):959-60.
81. Liu J, Tan L, Thigpen B, et al. Evaluation of the learning curve and safety outcomes in robotic assisted vaginal natural orifice transluminal endoscopic hysterectomy: a case series of 84 patients. Int J Med Robot. 2022:18(3):e2385.
82. Liu J. Surgical complications associated with laparoscopic myomectomy. Gynecol Surg. 2015;12(2):121-6.
83. Liu L, Li Y, Xu H, et al. Laparoscopic transient uterine artery occlusion and myomectomy for symptomatic uterine myoma. Fertil Steril. 2011;95(1):254-8.
84. Magrina JF. Laparoscopic versus open myomectomy: a systematic review. J Minim Invasive Gynecol. 2019;26(6):1006-14.
85. Management of Symptomatic Uterine Leiomyomas: ACOG Practice Bulletin, Number 228. Obstet Gynecol. 2021;137(6):e100-e15.
86. Martinez MEG, Domingo MVC. Size, type, and location of myoma as predictors for successful laparoscopic myomectomy- a tertiary government hospital experience. Gynecol Minim Invasive Ther. 2018;7(2):61-5.
87. Mason N. Obesity as a risk factor for complications in laparoscopic surgery. Surg Obes Relat Dis. 2020;16(2):187-94.
88. Mazzon I, Favilli A, Cocco P, et al. Does cold loop hysteroscopic myomectomy reduce intrauterine adhesions? A retrospective study. Fertil Steril. 2014;101(1): 294-8.e3.
89. Milad MP, Milad EA. Laparoscopic morcellator-related complications. J Minim Invasive Gynecol. 2014;21(3):486-91.
90. Miller CE, Wechter ME. 2015. Complications of laparoscopic myomectomy. Clin Obstetr Gynecol. 2015;58(1):91-113.
91. Moda N, Das S, Patro M, et al. Comparison of hemodynamic status and complications between two different doses of intramyometrial vasopressin during laparoscopic myomectomy: a retrospective study, the lesser the better. Asian J Pharm Clin Res. 2021;14(10):111-3.
92. Moen MD, Nothnick WB. Post-hysterectomy care: optimizing patient outcomes. J Minim Invasive Gynecol, 2023;30(3):433-40.
93. Mothes AR, Kather A, Cepraga I, et al. Robotic-assisted Gynecological Surgery in Older Patients—a Comparative Cohort Study of Perioperative Outcomes. Geburtshilfe Frauenheilkd. 2023;83(4):437-45.
94. Mourad A, Kamga-Ngande C, Albaini O, et al. Enhancing surgical performance: the role of robotic surgery in myomectomies, a systematic review and metanalysis. J Robot Surg. 2024;18(1):184.
95. Nagai A. Revised PREoperative sarcoma score for preoperative risk stratification of uterine sarcomas. Gynecol Oncol. 2018;149(1):92-8.
96. Nagai T, Takai Y, Akahori T, et al. Highly improved accuracy of the revised PREoperative sarcoma score (rPRESS) in the decision of performing surgery for patients presenting with a uterine mass. Springerplus. 2015;4:520.
97. Nensi A, Yeung GW, Frecker H, et al. Measures to reduce perioperative and intraoperative blood loss at myomectomy: A survey of obstetrician-gynaecologists. J Obstetr Gynaecol Can. 2020;42(5):550-5.
98. Neuwirth RS, Amin HK. Excision of submucus fibroids with hysteroscopic control. Am J Obstet Gynecol. 1976;126:95-9.

99. Nobbenhuis MAE, Gul N, Barton-Smith P, et al. Robotic surgery in gynaecology. BJOG. 2022;130(1):e1-e8.
100. Ozceltik G, Hortu I, Itil IM, et al. Vaginal approach versus laparoscopy for hysterectomy in transgender men. J Gynecol Obstet Hum Reprod. 2022;51(2): 102286.
101. Papadopoulos NP, Magos A. First-generation endometrial ablation: roller-ball vs loop vs laser. Best Prac Res Clin Obstetr Gynaecol. 2007;21(6):915-29.
102. Paredes JS, Lee CL, Chua PT. Myomectomy: Choosing the surgical approach: a systematic review. Gynecol Minim Invasive Ther. 2024;13:146-53.
103. Park SJ, Kim HS, Yim GW. Comparison of vaginal natural orifice transluminal endoscopic surgery (vNOTES) and laparoendoscopic single-site (LESS) hysterectomy on postoperative pain reduction: a randomized pilot study. Pain Ther. 2021;10(2):1401-11.
104. Park SJ, Lee JW, Hwang DW, et al. Effect and Safety of Diluted Vasopressin Injection for Bleeding Control During Robot-assisted Laparoscopic Myomectomy in Reproductive Women With Uterine Fibroids: A Randomized Controlled Pilot Trial (VALENTINE Trial). In Vivo. 2024;38(1):431-6.
105. Pelosi MA III, Pelosi MA. Laparoscopic-assisted transvaginal myomectomy. J Am Assoc Gynecol Laparosc. 1997;4:241-6.
106. Pickett CM, Seeratan DD, Mol BWJ, et al. Surgical approach to hysterectomy for benign gynaecological disease', Cochrane Database of Syst Rev. 2023;(8): CD003677.
107. Pisat S, van Herendael B. Pisat's Visual Vasopressor Injection Needle: An Innovative Tool for Increasing Patient Safety in Laparoscopic Myomectomy. Surg Technol Int. 2017;30;197-204.
108. Pisat S, van Herendael BJ. Temporary ligation of the uterine artery at its origin using a removable "shoelace" knot. J Minim Invasive Gynecol. 2020;27(1):26.
109. Pisat SV. Pisat's visual vasopressor injection needle: a new device for increasing patient safety in laparoscopic myomectomy. J Obstetr Gynecol India. 2017;67: 451-3.
110. Powers RD. Imaging modalities in the diagnosis of uterine fibroids. Ultrasound Obstet Gynecol. 2018;52(1):17-23.
111. Practice Committee of the American Society for Reproductive Medicine. Removal of myomas in asymptomatic patients to improve fertility and reduce miscarriage rate: a guideline. Fertil Steril. 2017; 108:416-25.
112. Pritts EA, Parker WH, Olive D. Fibroids and infertility : An updated systematic review of the evidence. Fertil Steril. 2009;91:1215-23.
113. Pritts EA, Parker WH, Olive D. Fibroids and infertility : An updated systematic review of the evidence. Fertil Steril. 2009;91:1215-23.
114. Pritts EA, Vanness DJ, Berek JS, et al. The prevalence of occult leiomyosarcoma at surgery for presumed uterine fibroids: a meta-analysis. Gynecol Surg. 2015; 12:165-77.
115. Protopapas A, Kathopoulis N, Chatzipapas I, et al. Misoprostol vs vasopressin as a single hemostatic agent in laparoscopic myomectomy: Comparable, or just better than nothing? J Obstetr Gynaecol Res. 2020;46(11), pp.2356-2365.
116. Raffi F. The role of blood work in patients with uterine fibroids. Eur J Obstet Gynecol Reprod Biol. 2020;250:173-7.

117. Rivard C, Salhader A, Kenton K. New challenges in detecting, grading, and staging endometrial cancer after uterine morcellation. J Minim Invasive Gynecol. 2012;19(3):313-6.
118. Rosen AD. Periareolar closure with barbed sutures. Aesthet Surg J. 2016; 36(3):372-5.
119. Royal College of Obstetricians and Gynaecologists. (2015). Obtaining a valid consent, Clinical Governance Advice No. 6. [online] Available from https://www.rcog.org.uk/guidance/browse-all-guidance/clinical-governance-advice/obtaining-valid-consent-clinical-governance-advice-no-6/ [Last accessed November, 2024].
120. Seidman JD. Morcellation of uterine tissue: a review of the literature. Fertil Steril. 2012;98(5):1075-80.
121. Sheng Y, Hong Z, Wang J, et al. Efficacy and safety of robot-assisted laparoscopic myomectomy versus laparoscopic myomectomy: a systematic evaluation and meta-analysis. World J Surg Oncol. 2023;21(1):230.
122. Sinai Talaulikar V, Belli AM, Manyonda I. GnRH agonists: do they have a place in the modern management of fibroid disease? J Obstet Gynaecol India. 2012; 62(5):506-10.
123. Sinha A, Pathak M, Vig A, et al. Robotic surgery in paediatric patients: Our initial experience and roadmap for successful implementation of robotic surgery programme. J Mini Access Surg. 2021;17(1):32-6.
124. Sinha R, Rupa B, Reddy M. Beyond the learning curve: improving outcomes in Robotic myomectomy compared to laparoscopic myomectomy. J Robot Surg. 2023;17(3):847-52.
125. Sinha R. Contained versus uncontained morcellation: a review of outcomes. Fertil Steril. 2019;111(6):1172-80.
126. Sleiman Z, El Baba R, Garzon S, et al. The significant risk factors of intra-operative hemorrhage during laparoscopic myomectomy: a systematic review. Gynecol Minim invasive Ther. 2020;9(1):6-12.
127. Smith M. Cost considerations in laparoscopic morcellation techniques. Gynecol Surg. 2021;18(1):1-8.
128. Soliman R, Yacoub A, Elbiaa AA. Assessment of the perioperative effect of vasopressin in patients undergoing laparoscopic myomectomy: A double-blind randomised study. Indian J Anaesth. 2021;65(2):139-45.
129. Sunkara SK, Khairy M, El-Toukhy T, et al. The effect of intramural fibroids without uterine cavity involvement on the outcome of IVF treatment: a systematic review and meta-analysis. Hum Reprod. 2010;25(2):418-29.
130. Tanos V, Berry KE, Frist M, et al. Prevention and management of complications in laparoscopic myomectomy. BioMed Res Int. 2018;(1):8250952.
131. Tanos V, Lee SC, Alexander K, et al. Laparoscopic myomectomy complications: Meta-analysis on RCTs and review of large cohort studies. Eur J Obstetr Gynecol Reprod Biol. 2023;287:109-18.
132. Tinelli A, Favilli A, Lasmar RB, et al. The importance of pseudocapsule preservation during hysteroscopic myomectomy. Eur J Obstet Gynecol Reprod Biol. 2019;243:179-84.
133. Topcu EG, McClenahan P, Pule K, et al. FIGO best practice guidance in surgical consent. Intl J Gynecol Obstetr. 2023;163(3):795-812.

134. Toubia T, Moulder JK, Schiff LD, et al. Peritoneal Washings After Power Morcellation in Laparoscopic Myomectomy: A Pilot Study. J Minim Invasive Gynecol. 2016;23(4):578-81.
135. van Dongen H, Emanuel MH, Wolterbeek R, et al. Hysteroscopic morcellator for removal of intrauterine polyps and myomas: a randomized controlled pilot study among residents in training. J Minim Invasive Gynecol. 2008;15: 466-547.
136. Van Wessel S, van Vliet H, Schoot BC, et al. Hysteroscopic morcellation versus bipolar resection for removal of type 0 and 1 submucous myomas: A randomized trial. EJOG. 2021;259:32-7.
137. Walters MD, Ferrando C, Sharp HT, et al. Hysterectomy (benign indications): Selection of surgical route. In: Post TW (ed.) UpToDate. Waltham, MA: UpToDate Inc.; 2024.
138. Wang C, Yen C, Lee C, et al. Laparoscopic-assisted vaginal myomectomy. J Am Assoc Gynecol Laparosc. 2000;7:510-4.
139. Wang CJ, Yuen LT, Han CM, et al. A transient blocking uterine perfusion procedure to decrease operative blood loss in laparoscopic myomectomy. Chang Gung Med J. 2008;31(5):463-8.
140. Wang T, Tang H, Xie Z, et al. Robotic-assisted vs. laparoscopic and abdominal myomectomy for treatment of uterine fibroids: A meta-analysis. Minim Invasive Ther Allied Technol. 2018;27(5):249-64.
141. Wong SW, Crowe P. Visualisation ergonomics and robotic surgery. J Robot Surg. 2023;17(5):1873-8.
142. Wu CZ, Klebanoff JS, Tyan P, et al. Review of strategies and factors to maximize cost-effectiveness of robotic hysterectomies and myomectomies in benign gynecological disease. J Robot Surg. 2019;13(5):635-42.
143. Wu PC, Sheu BC, Huang KJ, et al. Laparoendoscopic two-site myomectomy (LETS-M) using conventional laparoscopic instruments and the glove-port technique. J Formos Med Assoc. 2022;121(11):2248-56.
144. Yang WH, Luo N, Ma L, et al. The changes of surgical treatment for symptomatic uterine myomas in the past 15 years. Gynecol Minim Invasive therapy. 2018;1: 10-5.
145. Yin X, Cheng J, Ansari S, et al. Hysteroscopic tissue removal systems for the treatment of intrauterine pathology: a systematic review and meta-analysis. Facts Views Vis Ob Gyn. 2018:10;207-13.
146. Yoshiki N. Review of transvaginal natural orifice transluminal endoscopic surgery in gynecology. Gynecol Minim Invasive Ther. 2017;6(1):1-5.

CHAPTER 9

Alternative Modalities for Management of Fibroids

Suyash Naval, Poushali Sanyal

Q1. What are the alternate non-surgical methods for managing fibroids? *(Refer to section VII for medical treatment)*

Draft recommendations:

The nonsurgical methods are as follows:

- Uterine artery embolization (UAE)
- Magnetic resonance guided focused ultrasound surgery (MRgFUS) and high-intensity focused ultrasound (HIFU)
- *Ablation techniques:* Like Radiofrequency Ablation (RFA) and Microwave Ablation (MWA) or Percutaneous Microwave Ablation (PMWA).

UAE is a minimally invasive procedure that involves occlusion of uterine arteries bilaterally using particulate emboli resulting in ischemic necrosis of fibroids and thereby improving the associated symptoms.

MRgFUS is a noninvasive procedure that uses high intensity ultrasound waves to destroy fibroids without the need for surgery. The tissue is ablated through thermal and cavitation effects that result in destruction of the parenchymal and vascular endothelial cells of the tumor.

MEA involves the use of microwaves to heat and destroy the fibroid tissue. A thin needle-like probe is inserted into the fibroid, and microwaves are directed through the probe to heat and destroy the tissue. It is done under local anesthesia and guided by imaging techniques such as ultrasound.

RFA works in a similar way but uses radio-frequency energy instead of microwave to destroy tissue.

Review of literature: *The effective volume reduction in MRgFUS depends mainly on size and localization of the fibroids and achieved NPV (Non-perfused volume) ratio.*

Both MEA and RFA are effective, safe and have a shorter recovery time compared to traditional surgical procedures for fibroid management.

Q2. How are fibroid cases for ablation techniques chosen?

Draft recommendations: Fibroid cases for ablation are typically chosen based on several factors, including the size, location, and number of fibroids, as well as the patient's symptoms and overall health. Ablation is often considered for women who have symptomatic uterine fibroids, wish to avoid hysterectomy, and also have wishes for future fertility.

If the fibroid is intracavitary (not subserous or pedunculated), or it is a solitary fibroid less than 10 cm in diameter, then ablation of fibroids can be done.

If the woman has certain medical conditions that are a contraindication to invasive surgery under anesthesia, these alternative modalities are extremely beneficial.

Review of literature: *If the woman has symptomatic fibroids resulting in heavy periods, severe cramping, increased frequency of urination, and pelvic pain and pain during sex but wishes to retain her uterus, she is a good candidate for fibroid ablation. In some cases, a healthcare provider may also consider factors such as the patient's desire for future fertility, the presence of other medical conditions, and the potential risks and benefits of the procedure. Ultimately the decision to undergo fibroid ablation is individualized and based on a thorough evaluation of the patient's specific circumstances.*

Q3. What are the short and long term outcomes of ablation techniques?

Draft recommendations: The short term outcomes typically include immediate relief of symptoms such as menorrhagia, pelvic pain and pressure symptoms. Patients may experience a decrease in the size of their fibroids and improvement in the quality of life within a few weeks to months after the procedure.

Long-term outcomes after fibroid ablation techniques show that majority of patients experienced sustained relief of symptoms and improvement in quality of life for 5 years.

However, fibroids can sometimes recur, especially in younger patients or those with larger fibroids. In such cases, reintervention is necessary.

Review of literature: *Studies by Andersen in 2009 show that more than 90% of patients treated with ablation techniques had immediate relief of symptoms such as reduced bleeding, reduced pain and reduced pressure symptoms. At 6 to 12 months of treatment, the satisfaction rate and relief rate was 68%. Even after 5 years follow up, significant symptom relief was observed.*

Q4. What are the indications and contraindications of uterine artery embolization?

Draft recommendations: Indications of UAE are:

- Symptomatic intracavitary fibroids causing Heavy Menstrual Bleeding
- Pelvic pain or pressure due to fibroid growth
- Anemia caused by heavy menstrual bleeding due to uterine fibroids
- Desire to avoid surgery

Contraindications to UAE include:

- Pregnancy
- Active pelvic infection
- Severe coagulopathy
- Allergy to the contrast dye
- Severe renal impairment
- Active severe liver disease
- Severe arterial disease in the legs
- Large fibroids that may not respond well to embolization.

It is important for patients to discuss their medical history and any potential contraindications with their healthcare provider before undergoing UAE.

Review of literature: *The decision as to whether UAE is appropriate for a patient is based on a multilayered consideration of factors. Current pregnancy or active liver and renal disease, uncontrolled bleeding disorders are some of the conditions that are contraindications to the use of UAE as a treatment modality. Subserous pedunculated fibroids cannot be treated by UAE. Symptomatic intracavitary fibroids causing menorrhagia, anemia and bulk symptoms respond well to UAE.*

Q5. How does uterine artery embolization affect future fertility?

Draft recommendations: The potential implications for UAE on future fertility are as follows:

- *Reduced fertility:* The potential decrease in blood flow to the uterus can cause decreased chance of implantation of the embryo.
- *Increased risk of pregnancy complications:* In a pregnancy following UAE, there is a risk of placental abnormalities, preterm birth and miscarriage.
- Increased chance of Caesarean Section in future pregnancies.

Review of literature: *Studies by Bruce Mc Lucus et al. in 2019 have shown that there is negative impact of UAE on future fertility including delayed fertility. However, data is limited. Studies by Anneveldt KJ (2021) have shown that after UAE, pregnancy rates are low and miscarriage rates are higher than the baseline population. Women undergoing UAE also have a higher incidence of preterm births, placenta previa and Caesarean Sections.*

Q6. What is the current role of HIFU in fibroid management?

Draft recommendations:

- *US-guided HIFU treatment in patients with uterine fibroids is an effective therapeutic option which can be considered safe in an interdisciplinary setting.*

- *Analgesic treatment and body temperature management are critical points where an adequate cooperation of the intervention team is mandatory.*
- *More studies as well as innovative approaches are necessary to optimize peri-and postprocedural pain therapy.*

Discussion and review of literature: US-guided high-intensity-focused ultrasound (HIFU) and magnetic resonance-guided HIFU ablation treatment are now a new noninvasive surgical procedure that developed rapidly, with vast clinical experience accumulating in treating uterine fibroids, adenomyosis, and other gynecological diseases. HIFU ablation fibroid treatment is to focus US energy on a target point inside the fibroid; the energy can generate thermal heat up to 65–85°C and lead to coagulative necrosis without a cut wound.

This minimally invasive fibroid treatment has a high success rate of 90% in reducing the sizes and symptoms of fibroids. Vast clinical experience has been accumulated in treating uterine fibroids.

Unlike traditional surgery, in which wounds are made, with bleeding occurring and possible complications arising. The complications of the HIFU ablation procedure are mild, and the surrounding tissues and organs will often not be seriously damaged or injured. However, thermal injury to its surrounding organs has been reported, though they are few if properly performed by well-trained, experienced doctors.

As HIFU is a new treatment modality, accreditation and training programs have been proposed and developed to ensure its operation with high effectiveness and safety.

Q7. What is the current role of radio frequency ablation and microwave ablation for fibroid management?

Draft recommendations:

- *Radiofrequency ablation and microwave ablation can be considered as a micro-invasive treatment option in patients who desire to retain their uterus.*
- *The evidence on the safety of radiofrequency ablation and microwave ablation raises no major safety concerns, evidence on the efficacy of the procedure is limited in quality.*
- *The patients must be informed about the limited data on reproductive outcomes.*
- *There is no difference in the effectiveness of laparoscopic, transvaginal, or transcervical approaches using ultrasound guidance.*

Discussion and review of literature: RFA uses a high-frequency alternating electric current to induce focal ionic agitation around the probe tips with resultant rapid heat generation in the target tissues. The RFA procedure involves two approaches for treating fibroids: (1) using transvaginal US to locate the fibroids, an insulated RFA electrode is inserted through a very small abdominal incision to penetrate deep within the fibroid without harming surrounding tissue and (2) using transabdominal US to monitor the transcervical, intrauterine insertion of the insulated RFA shaft into the fibroid.

This procedure uses high heat to ablate fibroid tissue in a controlled thermal zone. Bradley et al. *(2019)* reviewed 32 articles of 1283 patients treated with laparoscopic and transvaginal RFA; they concluded that RFA of uterine fibroids significantly reduced fibroid volume (66%), improved quality of life (QOL), and was associated with favorable reintervention rates (4.2–11.5% in 3-year follow-up). RFA fibroids treatment has proven safe, easy to apply, and effective in reducing symptoms of uterine fibroids.

RFA has sometimes been limited by the lack of accurate monitoring of the ablated tissue zone, the precise location of fibroids by US imaging, and the need for multiple serosal punctures for multiple fibroids, leading to serosal injury, adhesions, and potential myometrial disruption during pregnancy.

Microwave is a heat-based ablation method, with cell death after exposure to elevated high temperature through the production of electromagnetic waves with resultant oscillation of water molecules within the target tissue. MWA has advantages over RFA, with a more rapid and sustained rise in temperature, good tissue penetration, and minimal heat sink effects when treating fibroids.

During WMA, the electrode antenna is accurately inserted into the fibroid under transabdominal US guidance. The microwave generator emits an electromagnetic wave with a frequency of 2450 MHz causing thermal necrosis. Ierardi et al. (2018) reviewed six papers using PubMed databases and reported the literature's overall experience of percutaneous MWA. Five hundred and forty-one patients (with 647 fibroids) were treated. The volume reduction rate of fibroids was from 15.9 to 93.1%, and the QOL improved after treatment. From these studies, US-guided percutaneous MWA is minimally invasive, has a short treatment duration, is easy to perform, and has been broadly used for the treatments of fibroids with favorable effects. There were no major complications requiring further interventions or hospitalization. Minor complications were observed, in particular lower abdominal pain, blood-stained vaginal discharge, and fragments of necrotic tissues from the vagina in some patients.

However, given the great variations in fibroid volume reduction, more cohort studies and randomized, prospective clinical trials are still needed to demonstrate the benefits of MWA in managing uterine fibroids.

Q8. What is the potential of using herbal supplements or dietary changes as alternative treatments for fibroids?

Draft recommendations:

- *Uterine fibroid risk is highly linked to vitamin D insufficiency. Insufficient vitamin D can cause cell proliferation and leiomyoma. Physiological vitamin D concentrations suppress fibroid cell development, especially in hypovitaminosis D individuals.*
- *There is no uniform consensus about the impact of vitamin A on uterine fibroids. A diet rich in carotenoids, such as lycopene, can reduce the incidence of uterine fibroids and promote decrease in volume.*
- *The role of vitamin C and E to treat uterine fibroids is unclear.*
- *A diet rich in fruits and vegetables, which contain carotenoids, quercetin, and indole-3-carbinol, may be one of the easiest and most effective lifestyle adjustments for women having leiomyoma. EGCG (epigallocatechin-3-gallate) and green tea extract may prevent and treat uterine fibroids.*
- *Curcumin, a natural substance with proven therapeutic effects on uterine fibroids, can reduce oxidative stress and protect against inflammation.*
- *The recommendation of dairy products (yogurt) and selenium having a beneficial effect on uterine fibroid related symptoms can be considered as weak.*

Discussion and review of literature: A comprehensive review of the literature published in the last 20 years about the relationship between dietary variables and the incidence of uterine fibroids (UFs) gives important insights to answer this question.

There is considerable evidence suggesting a connection between vitamin D deficiency and the growth of UFs, which makes vitamin D a powerful ingredient in the treatment of leiomyomas. Compounds similar to 25-hydroxyvitamin D3, which are not easily broken down by tissue 24-hydroxylase, show great potential and tend to yield improved therapeutic outcomes. Vitamin D3 activates the nuclear vitamin D receptor to perform its biological functions. Insufficient vitamin D3 causes uncontrolled proliferation, fibrosis, and chronic inflammation by activating fibroid cell development, damaged DNA, and reduced DNA repairability.

While there is conflicting information on the exact role of vitamin A in the development of fibroids, consuming a diet rich in vitamin A or using synthetic retinoid analogues may potentially prevent or restrict the growth of fibroids. Antioxidant carotenoids may lower uterine leiomyoma risk. He et al. found that premenopausal women who ate fiber- and lycopene-rich fruits and vegetables had a lower risk of fibroids than postmenopausal women.

Definitive findings cannot be made regarding the effectiveness of vitamin E and C supplementation, save for alpha-tocopherol. Alpha-tocopherol, a phytoestrogen that has a role in the regulation of estrogen receptors (ERs) implicated in the development of uterine fibroids, should be specifically avoided in treatment. Dietary vitamin E has no hazards, according to Wise et al. (2011). Vitamin E, despite its antioxidant characteristics, does not appear to prevent or treat leiomyoma.

A diet that contains a high amount of fruits and vegetables, which are rich in carotenoids, polyphenols, quercetin, and indole-3-carbinol, is a lifestyle factor that may be readily changed and has positive effects for patients with UFs.

Green tea is consumed worldwide for its antioxidant properties, notably in Asia. Its catechin content is higher than other drinks. Green tea contains polyphenols, flavones, and flavanols (kaempferol, myricetin, quercetin). In cultures of human uterine leiomyoma cells, EGCG in green tea extract reduced proliferation and growth and induced apoptosis dose-dependently. EGCG's antiproliferative and gene-modulating actions were partly modulated by COMT enzyme activity. Roshdy et al. (2013) found oral green tea extract (EGCG) safe and beneficial for symptomatic uterine fibroids. Many patients improved their health-related quality of life after taking 800 mg/day of EGCG, which reduced tumor volume and fibroid-specific symptoms. The European Food Safety Authority (EFSA) warns of hepatotoxic effects from using ≥800 mg EGCG/day as a dietary supplement.

Curcumin, along with other natural compounds, has the ability to decrease oxidative stress and provide protection against inflammation in leiomyoma. Curcumin is one of the three major curcuminoids in turmeric plant (*Curcuma longa*). Malik et al. (2009) demonstrated in vitro that curcumin inhibited the proliferation of uterine leiomyoma cells. The curcumin compound caused upregulation of the apoptotic pathway and inhibited fibronectin production, a component of ECM. Indole-3-carbinol (I3C) and quercetin, plant-derived components, were also considered UF treatments.

Q9. Can acupuncture or traditional Chinese medicine help alleviate symptoms associated with fibroids?

Draft recommendations: *Uterine fibroids may be treated conservatively with acupuncture, which has demonstrated promise.*

Research gap: Additional rigorous randomized controlled trials and extended follow-up studies are necessary to further validate the efficacy and safety of acupuncture in the treatment of uterine fibroids.

Discussion and review of literature: TCM (Traditional Chinese Medicine)-based acupuncture has been utilized for thousands of years to treat many illnesses. Acupuncture is less intrusive and has few negative effects when done by a professional. By controlling GnRH and other reproductive hormones, acupuncture regulates the HPO axis. Local blood flow modification is another possibility. Acupuncture increases blood flow to the uterus and surrounding tissues. Increased blood flow may lessen uterine fibroid size and symptoms. Uterine fibroid acupuncture treatment is viable and has no major side effects, according to early studies. Subgroup meta-analysis indicates that electroacupuncture and traditional acupuncture reduce fibroids or uterus volume more effectively than conventional treatment after 1–3 months of treatment. Subgroup analysis of alternative acupuncture treatments for uterine fibroids and long-term efficacy is not possible due to a lack of high-quality data.

According to Liu S et al. (2022), acupuncture can promote microcirculation and suppress excessive fibrosis, which may treat uterine fibroids. However, few clinical investigations have not conclusively shown that acupuncture treats uterine fibroids. A systematic database evaluation found 11 randomized controlled studies and provided higher-quality evidence for acupuncture treatment of uterine fibroids. Each study employed uterine fibroid or uterine volume as a therapeutic index, demonstrating that Chinese patients and clinicians want to reduce UF volume. In about half of the studies, patients with TCM syndrome differentiation were recruited or differentiated during acupuncture point selection, indicating that acupuncture, a classic TCM treatment method, is related to disease types and syndrome types. However, more research is needed to discover if syndrome differentiation benefits myoma patients. Also, uterine fibroids require estrogen. Western medicine treats UFs by reducing estrogen, which reduces myoma size. Still, acupuncture cannot reduce estrogen, which may prove that TCM treats fibroids differently from Western medicine and that the specific molecular pathways affected by acupuncture need further experimental research. Uterine fibroid therapy with acupuncture is safe, according to studies. The normal blood, liver, and renal function in all trials can help ensure participant safety. There are some limitations with the current data. Traditional, electro, heated, and moxibustion acupuncture procedures, frequency, and course of treatment vary. These factors can impact effect measurement and cause heterogeneity. Second, part of the design of experiments is incomplete, such as the acupuncture operation and the researcher's background, which limits our evaluation of the literature.

BIBLIOGRAPHY

1. Andersen PE, Lund N. Uterine artery embolisation of symptomatic uterine fibroids: Initial Success and short-term results. Acta Radiologica. 2009;42(2): 234-8.
2. Anneveldt KJ, van 't Oever HJ, Nijholt IM, et al. Systematic review of reproductive outcomes after high intensity focused ultrasound treatment of uterine fibroids. Eur J Radiol. 2021;141:109809.

3. Brace CL. Microwave ablation technology: What every user should know. Curr Probl Diagn Radiol. 2009;38:61-7.
4. Bradley LD, Pasic RP, Miller LE. Clinical performance of radiofrequency ablation for treatment of uterine fibroids: Systematic review and meta-analysis of prospective studies. J Laparoendosc Adv Surg Tech A. 2019;29:1507-17.
5. Chang R, Chung PH, Rosenwaks Z. Role of acupuncture in the treatment of female infertility. Fertil Steril. 2002;78:1149-53.
6. Chen J, Li Y, Wang Z, et al. Evaluation of high-intensity focused ultrasound ablation for uterine fibroids: An IDEAL prospective exploration study. BJOG. 2018;125:354-64.
7. EFSA Panel on Food Additives and Nutrient Sources added to Food (ANS); Younes M, Aggett P, Aguilar F, et al. Scientific opinion on the safety of green tea catechins. EFSA J. 2018;16:e05239.
8. He Y, Zeng Q, Dong S, et al. Associations between uterine fibroids and lifestyles including diet, physical activity and stress: A case-control study in China. Asia Pac. J. Clin. Nutr. 2013;22:109-17.
9. Hwang DW, Song HS, Kim HS, et al. Delayed intestinal perforation and vertebral osteomyelitis after high-intensity focused ultrasound treatment for uterine leiomyoma. Obstet Gynecol Sci. 2017;60:490-3.
10. Liu L, Wang T, Lei B. Uterine artery embolization compared with high intensity focused ultrasound ablation for the treatment of symptomatic uterine myomas : A systemic review and meta analysis. JMIG. 2020;28;218-27.
11. Liu W, Wang CC, Lee KH, et al. Research methodology in acupuncture and moxibustion for managing primary dysmenorrhea: a scoping review. Complement Ther Med. 2022;71:102874.
12. Liu Y, Zhang WW, He M, et al. Adverse effect analysis of high intensity focused ultrasound in the treatment of benign uterine diseases. Int J Hyperthermia. 2018;35:56-1.
13. Malik M, Mendoza M, Payson M, et al. Curcumin, a nutritional supplement with antineoplastic activity, enhances leiomyoma cell apoptosis and decreases fibronectin expression. Fertil. Steril. 2009;91:2177-84.
14. McLucas B, Elliott S, Elliott S. Fertility after Uterine artery Embolisation: a review. Minim Invasive Ther Allied Technol. 2015;25(1):1-7.
15. Spies JB. Uterine Artery Embolisation - Indications and Contraindications. In: Reidy, J, Hacking N, McLucus B (ed). Radiological Interventions in Obstetrics and Gynaecology. Medical Radiology. Berlin, Heidelberg: Springer; 2012.
16. Taheri M, Potts C, Quinn DS. Nonresective treatments for uterine fibroids: a systematic review of uterine and fibroid volume reductions. Int J Hyperth. 2019;36:294-300.
17. Wang L, Xu J, Yu J, et al. Review of clinical tumor ablation advance in Asia. Int J Hyperthermia. 2021;38:1639-49.
18. Wise LA, Radin RG, Palmer JR, et al. Intake of fruit, vegetables, and carotenoids in relation to risk of uterine leiomyomata. Am J Clin Nutr. 2011;94:1620-31.
19. Wong F, Zhang L, Wang Z. Focused Ultrasound Surgery in Gynecology: Introduction and Application. Singapore: Springer Nature; 2021.
20. Wong WS, Wong PH, Lee MH, et al. A proposed high intensity focused ultrasound training program in Hong Kong. Gynecol Minim Invasive Ther 2022;11:1-6.

21. Xu F, Deng L, Hu H, et al. The comparison of myomectomy, UAE and MRgFUS in the treatment of uterine fibroids: a meta-analysis. Int J Hyperth. 2021;38:24-9.
22. Zhang N, Rajaratnam V, Al-Hendy O, et al. Green Tea Extract Inhibition of Human Leiomyoma Cell Proliferation Is Mediated via Catechol-O-Methyltransferase. Gynecol Obstet Investig. 2014;78:109-18.
23. Zhu J, Li J, Yang L, et al. Acupuncture, from the ancient to the current. Anat Rec (Hoboken). 2021;304:2365-71.

CHAPTER 10

Risk of Malignancy in Fibroids

Bidisha Roychoudhury, Monika Anant, Tulika Jha

Q1. What is the incidence of malignant transformation in fibroids? What is the incidence of uterine leiomyosarcoma occurring de novo in women?

Draft recommendations:

- *Leiomyosarcomas are the most common uterine sarcomas, with an estimated annual incidence of 0.5–7/100,000 per women, followed by endometrial stromal sarcomas with an annual incidence of 1–2/million per women.*
- *Malignant leiomyosarcomas are rare and can arise de novo. The incidence of malignant degeneration is less than 1.0% and has been estimated to be as low as 0.2%.*

Summary of evidence: A genetic predisposition to leiomyoma growth exists. On the malignant spectrum, uterine sarcomas tend to occur in an older patient population when compared to leiomyomas, and only account for 3–7% of all uterine malignancies. Leiomyosarcomas are the most common uterine sarcomas, with an estimated annual incidence of 0.5–7/100,000 per women, followed by endometrial stromal sarcomas with an annual incidence of 1–2/million per women. The true incidence of malignant transformation is difficult to determine, because leiomyomas are common, whereas malignant leiomyosarcomas are rare and can arise de novo. The incidence of malignant degeneration is less than 1.0% and has been estimated to be as low as 0.2%.

Q2. What clinical symptoms or signs would make you suspicious for malignancy in fibroids?

Draft recommendations:

- *Symptoms arising from uterine disease are manifold and overlapping can manifest in severe pelvic pain, painful periods and non-cyclic pain, impaired fertility or outright infertility, fatigue, painful intercourse (dyspareunia), and bladder and bowel dysfunction (dysuria and dyschezia, respectively). Uterine fibroids in addition provoke heavy menstrual bleeding (HMB) as a prominent symptom in ~30% of patients and can further lead to feelings of pelvic pressure and bulging abdominal protuberances.*

- *Uterine STUMPs represent smooth-muscle tumors with equivocal histopathological features, insufficient for neither leiomyoma nor leiomyosarcoma diagnosis. Although they rarely prove to have a malignant behavior (e.g., recurrence, metastases), as malignancy cannot be excluded, these patients receive long-term imaging follow-up after surgical removal.*

Summary of evidence: Leiomyomas and Leiomyosarcomas have a very similar clinical presentation, although the mean age at presentation for leiomyosarcomas (45 years and greater) is usually higher than for leiomyomas (under 45 years). Women with these conditions can present with clinical symptoms such as profuse menstrual bleeding, pelvic discomfort, infertility, increased urinary frequency or incontinence, constipation and dyspareunia. Therefore, early distinction of leiomyosarcomas from a benign uterine leiomyoma can prove challenging clinically.

Q3. Association of fibroids with other gynecological diseases benign and malignant.

Draft recommendations:

- *The most common conditions to consider are adenomyosis, endometriosis, leiomyosarcoma, endometrial carcinoma and uterine carcinosarcoma.*
- *The genetic foundations of both uterine fibroids and endometriosis remain to be fully understood but recent evidence suggest common underpinnings.*

Summary of evidence: There is a frequent association between adenomyosis and other estrogen dependent benign diseases such as endometrial polyps, anovulation, hyperplasia, LM suggesting that hyperestrogenic state may share the common pathogenesis of these gynecological diseases and endometrial cancer. It has been found that annexin A2 is a key mediator in endometrial tissue growth, metastasis, and angiogenesis. p53 positivity was found in hyperplastic and atypical epithelia of carcinoma in adenomyotic patients.

Q4. What potential advancements in diagnostic techniques or biomarkers are available to help in early detection of malignancy in fibroids?

Draft recommendations:

- LDH and NLR are potentially useful markers in the diagnosis of a uterine sarcoma.
- Circulating biomarkers as a liquid biopsy could be beneficial as a diagnostic tool (proteins; circulating tumor cells; circulating tumor DNA; microRNA; and immune cells).
- *Molecular methods:* Leiomyomas are characterized by low expression of Ki-67, p53 and high expression of ER and PR receptors. In Leiomyosarcomas cell proliferation markers are increased (Ki67, p53). More evidence is necessary to better differentiate smooth muscle cell tumors.

Summary of evidence: Biomarkers from blood or body fluids can serve as potential markers for malignancy. In uterine sarcomas, most studied proteins are vascular endothelial growth factor (VEGF), basic fibroblast growth factor (bFGF), interleukins (IL), cancer antigen 125 (CA 125), lactate dehydrogenase, gangliosides (LDH) and growth differentiation factor 15 (GDF-15). LMP2/β1i and cyclin B1 have been studied in human uterine leiomyosarcoma.

Circulating biomarkers; such as proteins; circulating tumor cells; circulating tumor DNA; microRNA; and immune cells are also potential markers.

The blood-based liquid biomarkers that can be employed in clinical practice are lactate dehydrogenase (LDH), cancer-antigen 125 (CA125), and neutrophil-to-lymphocyte ratio (NLR). LDH and NLR are potentially useful markers in the diagnosis of a uterine sarcoma.

Q5. What imaging features are useful in differentiating leiomyoma from leiomyosarcoma?

Draft recommendations:

- No imaging modalities can definitively differentiate or rule out leiomyosarcoma. However in suspicion especially in high risk group that following may be helpful.
- A standardized sonographic approach to myometrial lesions should be always performed according to MUSA (morphological uterus sonographic assessment) criteria.
- On ultrasonography showing large size, degenerative cystic changes, and increased vascularity on color Doppler should raise suspicion of malignancy.
- CT scan detects calcifications present in leiomyomas as well as in Leiomyosarcomas.
- MRI is the preferred imaging modality for in-depth evaluation of myomas and for delineation of local spread of malignant disease.

Summary of evidence: The features on ultrasound for leiomyosarcoma are single, ≥8 cm fast-growing, oval/lobulated masses with inhomogeneous echogenicity, rarely with the fan-shaped shadowing, frequent areas of irregular cystic spaces signifying areas of central necrosis, frequently "Cooked" appearance and irregular vessels with score of 3–4.

On MRI, LMSs usually present as solitary heterogeneous and poorly demarcated masses. Areas of high signal intensity on T1-weighted images, corresponding to hemorrhage or necrosis, favoring malignancy. The highly cellular leiomyomas demonstrate marked early contrast enhancement. LMSs enhance early and heterogeneously, often demonstrating non-enhancing areas of central necrosis after gadolinium contrasts

Q6. What are the histopathological and cytogenetic features of leiomyoma versus leiomyosarcoma?

Draft recommendations:

- Histopathological criteria are increased mitotic index, cellular atypia, cellularity, and geographic areas of coagulative necrosis separated from viable neoplasm.
- Molecular-based diagnostics for leiomyosarcomas are present but no current clinical consensus exist.

Gross appearance would show loss of the typical whorl pattern, homogeneous texture, yellow color, soft consistency, absence of a bulging surface when the capsule is incised and having ill-defined margins on enucleation.

Appearance as a solitary, bulky, fleshy mass within the myometrium intramural (majority), submucosal, subserosal or pedunculated having hemorrhagic, necrotic and cystic areas. The average diameter is 10 cm, however about 25% are <5 cm. The myxoid leiomyosarcoma have gelatinous cut surface and are friable.

The essential histopathological diagnostic criteria require 2 of the 3 histologic features of marked cytologic atypia ≥10 mitoses/10 high power fields.

Tumor cell necrosis identified by abrupt transition from viable tumor cells to necrotic cells and the granulation tissue surrounding necrosis is absent.

Few cytogenetic features reported by few researches are the survivin, A transcriptomic analysis revealed 489 differentially expressed genes between these two conditions, as well as structural rearrangements targeting ATRX and RAD51B, overexpression of matrix metalloproteinase-14 (MMP14).

Q7. Can endometrial sampling predict sarcoma?

Draft recommendations: Endometrial sampling detects uterine sarcomas in only one-third–two-thirds patients but should be considered for patients for whom sarcoma is suspected by clinical and imaging characteristics and for whom myomectomy with intra-peritoneal morcellation is planned.

A preoperative diagnosis is achieved in only 33 to 68 percent of patients with uterine sarcomas by endometrial biopsy.

Q8. Is the frozen section recommended in suspicious cases?

Draft recommendations: Frozen section analysis intra-operatively can be done in high risk suspicious cases however it is not definitive and not reliable for excluding uterine sarcoma. So, it is not universally preferred or performed.

If it is done, the cellularity, significant cytologic atypia, number of unequivocal mitotic figures and tumor cell necrosis are to be assessed in the sample. The procedure of getting frozen section from multiple sites from the leiomyoma may lead to the diagnostic pitfall of not sampling the affected area. High chances of false. negative reporting can be there.

Q9. What are the lacunae or dilemmas in differentiating leiomyoma from leiomyosarcoma?

Research gaps: The main point of dilemmas for differentiating leiomyoma (ULM), especially the degenerated varieties, from leiomyosarcoma (ULMS) are the presence of similar clinical features and ultrasonography pictures. Computed tomography (CT) and MRI scans are more helpful in differentiating hyaline degeneration or necrosis from tumor necrosis. PET-CT scan is more useful in such cases. Endometrial biopsy is not of much help unless the mass is submucous.

There are quite a few therapeutic gaps, unmet medical needs and future perspectives especially in the areas of early and specific diagnosis.

Q10. What are the areas for future research and investigation into the molecular mechanisms underlying malignant transformation in fibroids?

The most important prognostic factor for uterine LMS is the extent of the disease at the time of diagnosis. The earlier the disease is diagnosed, the better the prognosis. Research is ongoing in multiple areas to facilitate early diagnosis and differentiation between ULM and ULMS.

Molecular features:

- *Role of endometrial biopsy:* The utility of endometrial biopsy in diagnosing ULMS is disputable but several studies have shown evidence which show more chances of detecting it when endometrial sampling is done along with hysteroscopy. When the results between dilatation and curettage and Pipelle's endometrial biopsy were compared, there was no statistically significant difference between the outcomes. Moreover, considering the low cost of both methods (biopsy, curettage) and the low risk of complications they may cause, their use in preoperative diagnostics seems justified.
- *Needle biopsy:* Transcervical needle biopsy from the suspicious uterine mass has been performed and the biopsy material, then, studied for degree of cellular atypia, mitotic index and coagulative necrosis. Immunohistochemical features were also studied namely CD34 (a protein expressed in early haemopoietic and vascular associated tissue), Ki-67 (a proliferation marker for human tumor cells) and a scoring system was used to calculate the score.

  Cases which have two or more positive factors (six or more points in the scale of 19 points) were classified as LMS. The positive predictive value, when the cut-off score was six points, was 100%, therefore it may become a very useful scoring system for cases that included a needle biopsy before surgery. But not all patients undergo needle biopsy and this is one area which can be studied in more details.

- *Circulating biomarkers:* New biomarkers namely growth differentiation factor 15 (GDF-15) and microRNA (miRNA) are being tested in blood to differentiate between ULM and ULMS. GDF-15, a divergent member of the TGF-β superfamily, is connected with the evolution of cancer and an especially high GDF-15 median levels can be seen in women with ULMS.

  Studies have also shown that two miRNAs, miR-1246 and miR-191-5p, may be one of the ULMS biomarkers, which could help in ULMS and ULM preoperative differentiation.
- In the scale of Nagai et al., named as the PREoperative Sarcoma Score (PRESS), they evaluated the utility of clinical findings, blood tests, imaging studies (USS and MRI) and endometrial cytology of 63 suspected uterine sarcoma cases. From all parameters, age, LDH, MRI and endometrial cytology findings were the most important predictors for sarcoma. In their seven-point system, two points were given in the cases of age ≥49, when the serum LDH values were ≥279 and where cytological findings were present. Furthermore, one point was for positive MRI finding. The authors used three points as a cut-off score—the patients with a score of three or higher should undergo surgery and those with two points or less could avoid it.
- *Radiomics and Artificial Intelligence (AI):* In recent years, a machine learning model is being used to differentiate between benign and malignant tumor. Three different volumes of interests (1) tumor; (2) tumor and small piece of surrounded tissue; and (3) whole uterus were analyzed using radiomics. The VOI radiomic model with the best diagnostic performance was the one that covered the whole uterus including the highest AUC, sensitivity, specificity and accuracy.

Q11. What would be the preferred surgery for suspicious masses: Hysterectomy or myomectomy?

Draft recommendations:

- *Total hysterectomy with bilateral salpingo-oophorectomy (TAH + BSO) is the surgery of choice in women with uterine masses.*
- *Salpingo-oophorectomy can be individualized in women in the reproductive age group but it should be preferred in women with positive ER/PR status.*
- *If the disease is unsuitable for primary surgery, plan for radiation therapy – pelvic External Beam Radiation Therapy (EBRT) with or without brachytherapy.*

- *When diagnosed after a myomectomy or TAH with BSO, patient may have to undergo surgery to remove all reproductive organs and any other resectable lesions and may need chemotherapy and radiotherapy.*

Summary of evidence: If the uterine leiomyoma (ULM) or mass is suspicious, surgery is indicated. The choice and extent of surgery will depend upon the pre-operative work up and diagnosis, the estrogen and progesterone receptor (ER/PR) status, the availability of frozen section biopsy, the age, reproductive planning and the wishes of the patient.

If uterine leiomyosarcoma (ULMS) or a STUMP is *diagnosed pre-operatively and the disease is limited to the uterus,* total hysterectomy with bilateral salpingo-oophorectomy is indicated. Salpingo-oophorectomy can be individualized in women in the reproductive age group but it should be preferred in women with positive ER/PR status. If there is additional discovery of an extra-uterine lesion during surgery, its resection needs to be individualized. Consider resection depending upon the extent of the disease and its resectability.

If the disease is *unsuitable for primary surgery,* plan for radiation therapy–pelvic External Beam Radiation Therapy (EBRT) with or without brachytherapy. Systemic therapy should also be considered in these women.

In most of the women, ULMS is diagnosed post-operatively following either a myomectomy or a total or subtotal hysterectomy with or without bilateral salpingo-oophorectomy.

When diagnosed after a myomectomy, a second expert pathologist's review opinion should be sought. Imaging namely USG or MRI or PET-CT scans should be done to find out the extent and spread of the disease along with an ER/PR status testing. If the diagnosis is confirmed as ULMS, a total hysterectomy with or without bilateral salpingo-oophorectomy should be done in cases where the disease is limited to the uterus. The rest of the management is as in the case of a pre-operatively diagnosed LMS.

In cases where LMS is diagnosed post-operatively following a total or subtotal hysterectomy with or without bilateral salpingo-oophorectomy, a second expert pathologist's review opinion should be sought. Imaging namely USG or MRI or PET-CT scans should be done to find out the extent and spread of the disease along with an ER/PR status testing. If the diagnosis of ULMS is confirmed, remove the residual cervix. Consider unilateral (in younger women) or bilateral salpingo-oophorectomy in ER/PR positive patients.

Q12. What is the survival rate of malignancy in fibroids?

The survival rate of uterine leiomyosarcoma mainly depends upon the extent of the disease at the time of diagnosis.

- Adnexal spread.
- Lymph node metastases.

- Tumor size.
- Peritoneal cytologic findings.
- Depth of myometrial invasion.

Factors that bear no relationship to the presence or absence of metastases at surgical exploration include the following:
- Presence or absence of stromal heterologous elements.
- Types of such elements.
- Grade of the stromal components.
- Mitotic activity of the stromal components.

The 5-year survival rates (according to the surveillance, epidemiology and end results (SEER) staging, are as follows.

SEER stage	***Survival rates LMS***	***Survival rates Undifferentiated sarcoma***
Localized	60%	71%
Regional	37%	37%
Distant	12%	18%
All SEER stages combined	38%	43%

BIBLIOGRAPHY

1. Choi EJ, Cho SB, Lee SR, et al. Comorbidity of gynecological and non-gynecological diseases with adenomyosis and endometriosis. Obstet Gynecol Sci. 2017;60:579.
2. David B Chapel 2022 Am J Surg Pathol Laganà AS et al. 2024 Gynecol Obstet Invest.
3. Del Carmen MG. Uterine leiomyosarcoma. In: del Carmen MG, Young RH, Schorge JO, Birrer MJ (Eds). Uncommon gynecologic cancers. India: Wiley-Blackwell; 2014.
4. Gonzalez-Molina J, Hahn P, Falcão RM, et al. MMP14 expression and collagen remodelling support uterine leiomyosarcoma aggressiveness. Mol Oncol. 2024;18(4):850-65.
5. Hinchcliff EM, Esselen KM, Watkins JC, et al. The Role of Endometrial Biopsy in the Preoperative Detection of Uterine Leiomyosarcoma. J Minim Invasive Gynecol. 2016;23(4):567-72.
6. Klaudia Z, Zaremba B, Rajtak A, et al. Preoperative Differentiation of Uterine Leiomyomas & Leiomyosarcomas: Current Possibilities and Future Direction. Cancers (Basel). 2022;14(8):1966.
7. Raffone A. A systematic review and meta-analysis. Int J Gynaecol Obstet. 2024.
8. Xie H, Hu J, Zhang X, et al. Preliminary utilization of radiomics in differentiating uterine sarcoma from atypical leiomyoma: Comparison on diagnostic efficacy of MRI features and radiomic features. Eur J Radiol. 2019;115:39-45.
9. Yokoi A, Matsuzaki J, Yamamoto Y, et al. Serum microRNA profile enables preoperative diagnosis of uterine leiomyosarcoma. Cancer Sci. 2019;110:3718-26.

CHAPTER 11

Psychological and Medicolegal Implications of Fibroids

Charu Mittal, Bidisha Roychoudhury

Q1. What are the potent psychological effects of fibroids on patients emotional wellbeing, economical impact, and quality of life?

Draft recommendations:

- *Fibroids significantly impact the quality of life (QOL) and mental health of affected women.*
- *Though they can cause a wide range of symptoms and infertility, fibroid treatment options remain limited. The fact that fibroids are under-discussed adds to the psychological stress of the women who carry them, Individuals with fibroids need to listen to their bodies and be proactive about discussing symptoms with a gynecologist.*
- *According to USA statistics approximately 200,000 hysterectomies and 30,000 myomectomies are performed for fibroid disease annually. When adjusted to 2023 USD, the economic burden is estimated to be $44 billion USD annually to the US healthcare system. In addition to healthcare costs, indirect costs due to disability and time taken off from work were estimated to be 1.55–17.2 billion 2010 USD annually.*

Notably, the QOL scores for uterine fibroids were similar to, or worse than, those associated with a diagnosis of diabetes mellitus, heart disease, or breast cancer. This reduction in the QOL in women with fibroids adversely impacts their mental health. Uterine fibroids are reported to be among the greatest psychological stressors for women, adversely affecting emotional and mental health determined by QOL measures, surveys, and semistructured interviews. Women affected with fibroids have 1.12-fold higher rates of depression and anxiety. Shen et al. found that the incidence of depression in women with uterine leiomyomas was 7.48 per 1,000 women vs. 4.88 per 1,000 without fibroids. Glover et al. conducted a survey in 200 women with fibroids in London and found that 35% of women scored in the borderline or clinical range for depression and 61% scored in the borderline or clinical range for anxiety. After adjusting for confounders, including a diagnosis of cancer, mental health condition, prescription for antidepressant medication, and age of 50 years before hysterectomy, patients with fibroids had higher rates of depression, anxiety, and self-directed violence.

The psychological distress secondary to fibroids does not end upon their removal, as the risk of regrowth is around 15-30 percent. As a result, multiple surgeries may be necessary. Waiting for regrowth after surgery, or more fibroid growth pre-surgery, can lead to anxiety and dread.

Q2. How do patients typically cope with psychological challenges associated with fibroids?

Draft recommendations:
- *Allowing herself to acknowledge the seriousness of fibroid*
- *Be the first person to acknowledge your own pain*
- *Contact a gynecologist immediately*
- *Form support groups amongst themselves to discuss and talk about their problems.*

Acknowledge the impact on life, even if society still has catching up to do. The worries about the impact of fibroids are valid and it is not easy to live waiting to see how they might further impact her functioning or fertility. Despite the impact of fibroids on women's lives, many women feel that they lack support to help them deal with these issues and very few seek help from a mental health professional. The Fibroid Foundation Organization is a global organization helping women all over the world.

Q3. What role do healthcare providers play in addressing the psychological needs of patients with fibroids?

Draft recommendations:
- Early response by healthcare providers to patients in distress
- Counseling patients to review for any menstrual complaints or pelvic pain
- There is an opportunity and a need for the mental health community to address the concerns in this population.

Leveraging the unique expertise and role of the mental health professional may lead to improved psychological health and quality of life in patients living with this chronic condition. Multidisciplinary team to be formed and advocated for management. Counseling groups and patient support groups to be encouraged, where they can discuss and share their concerns.

MEDICOLEGAL IMPLICATIONS OF FIBROIDS

INTRODUCTION

Considering the wide range of presentation of symptomatic as well as asymptomatic fibroids as well as their possible effects at different sites and the large treatment armamentarium available, as well as potential complications it is imperative for clinicians to be aware of the potential areas vulnerable to litigation.

Q4. Are there any legal implications related to the diagnosis or treatment of fibroids such as delayed diagnosis or mismanagement of fibroids, accidental undiagnosed leiomyosarcoma or malignancy?

Draft recommendations:

Diagnosis:

Delayed diagnosis is possible in young patients who approach for treatment of abnormal uterine bleeding where hormonal disorders are often considered as the common underlying cause and ultrasound may not be done in every patient.

Misdiagnosis: Identifying a Fibroid vs. Adenomyoma to decide proper management options. For example an adenomyoma causing subfertility may require a different approach in management compared to a fibroid and misdiagnosing one for the other can lead to difficulty in correct treatment.

Similarly, identification of leiomyosarcoma may not be possible pre-operatively and can lead to inappropriate surgical procedures like morcellation or delayed surgery which can worsen the prognosis of the patient.

Patients may be informed that the risk of unsuspected cancer increases with age particularly in women over 50 years of age, especially with fibroids larger than 5 cms. The USFDA estimates that a hidden uterine sarcoma may be present in approximately 1 in 225 to 1 in 580 women undergoing surgery for fibroids. The FDA also estimates that a leiomyosarcoma may be present in approximately 1 in 495 to 1 in 1100 women undergoing surgery for fibroids based on recent studies.

Treatment: Treatment options: medical, surgical, non-surgical - discussion about the advantages and limitations of chosen modality for treatment.

- *Medical management options:*
    - Available drugs like mifepristone, ulipristal acetate, cabergoline, GnRH analogs, DMPA, progesterone, tranexamic acid, OCPs, NSAIDs. Duration of use, potential side effects, chance of success as well as recurrence, possible need for surgery later, effect of medications on fertility.
    - *LNG IUD:* Pros and cons must be discussed
- *Surgical management options:*
    - *Myomectomy:* Discussion about routes - conventional/open, endoscopic (laparoscopic, hysteroscopic, Robotic) - feasibility, advantages/disadvantages, potential complications, sequelae (like recurrence, adhesions, subfertility, rarely upgradation of an undiagnosed uterine malignancy) and post-operative precautions relevant to procedure,

estimated cost involved. Appropriate Morcellation methods to be adopted prudently and tissue must be sent for pathological examination. US FDA May 26, 2023 recommendation states that laparoscopic power morcellation for myomectomy or hysterectomy be performed only with a tissue containment system. Consent must be obtained after explaining risk of parasitic fibroid development and inadvertent spread of a previously undiagnosed uterine malignancy. For individuals who are over 50 years of age or post-menopausal this procedure should not be recommended.

As of the late 2010 s and early 2020 s, in the United States, litigation related to power morcellators continues.

Patient needs to be advised and consent taken about occasional need for hysterectomy while performing a myomectomy. There is a wide range quoted for conversion of myomectomy to hysterectomy from as low as <0.1% up to 8%. Approximately 1–4% of open myomectomies may be converted to hysterectomy while 8% of laparoscopic myomectomies are converted to hysterectomy.

  - *Hysterectomy:* Routes—conventional/open, vaginal, laparoscopic, robotic

- *Non-surgical management options*: Advantages as well as limitations of each must be discussed
  - Uterine artery embolization (UAE)
  - *MRgFUS:* Magnetic resonance guided focused ultrasound surgery
  - USG-guided transcervical radiofrequency ablation (RFA)
  - Endometrial ablation (via laser/loop/balloon)

Q5. What are the medico-legal safeguards to be followed when dealing with a patient of fibroid?

Draft recommendations:

How to reduce risk for litigation?

- Detailed history taking and systematic examination to arrive at the correct diagnosis and to further tailor treatment options as per the patient profile.
- Investigations relevant to diagnosis and treatment. Prudent and justifiable use of Imaging modalities like ultrasound, MRI for location, number, size, mapping, vascularity, any other co-existing, incidental pathology to plan the treatment.
- Counseling of patient and relatives about the condition, available diagnostic modalities, natural history of the disorder, potential associated problems like subfertility, problems during pregnancy, abnormal uterine bleeding, pressure effects, recurrence after removal, remote risk of malignancy, etc., and available treatment options tailored to her clinical situation.

- Patient communication about available options with pros and cons of each treatment modality while keeping in mind her desire for fertility and conservative management.
- Using evidence-based guidelines and standard protocols in clinical practice as a fundamental issue to limit medico-legal responsibility
- Suggest a second opinion when decision making is difficult for the patient
- Referral to higher, better equipped center if limited facilities are available and patient is desirous of advanced treatment.
- Adequate training and supervision for selected procedure.
- Adequate Human and Equipment resources for selected procedure.
- Written, informed Consent for treatment mentioning the procedure planned, alternatives available, potential complications with incidence, additional procedures which may be required intra-operatively and consent preferably to be taken beforehand. Whichever treatment modality is chosen documentation of an accurate, pre-operative informed consent and refusal of treatment where applicable is a fundamental issue to limit medico-legal responsibility.
- Counseling must be done and consent must be taken pre-operatively for some specific situations which may occur during the surgery.
    - A proposed myomectomy may require conversion to a hysterectomy on table in approximately 1–4% of the cases.
    - A laparoscopic myomectomy may require intra-operative conversion to laparotomy in 8% of the procedures.

  All patients undergoing abdominal or laparoscopic myomectomies must be counseled about these above-mentioned possible complications when obtaining written, informed consent to reduce medico-legal liability.
- Safe and effective procedure following standard protocols. Prudent approach is to follow current recommendation to use a tissue containment system during power morcellation for myomectomy and hysterectomy both.
- Maintain treatment records especially intraoperative details, no discrepancy between documentation by involved consultants.
- Postoperative care and addressing complaints in a timely manner.
- Properly documented instructions and precautions at discharge
- Documentation of discussion at follow-up visit. Discussion of the further course of management especially if the histopathological report reveals that a presumed leiomyoma turned out to be a leiomyosarcoma.

BIBLIOGRAPHY

1. Dubuisson JB, Chapron C, Fauconnier A, et al. Laparoscopic myomectomy and myolysis. Curr Opin Obstet Gynecol. 1997;9:233-8.
2. Fersinil F, Maselli V, Miani E, et al. Misdiagnosis of leiomyosarcomas: case report and medico-legal issues. Gynecol Pelvic Med. 2021;4.

3. Leiomyoma Uterus/Fibromyoma/Fibroid Uterus. Standard Treatment Guidelines Obstetrics & Gynecology. Standard Treatment Guidelines—Speciality/Superspeciality wise. The Clinical Establishment Act 2010. India: MOHFW, GOI; 2010. pp. 5-12.
4. Olufowobi O, Sharif K, Papaionnou S, et al. Are the anticipated benefits of myomectomy achieved in women of reproductive age? a 5-year review of the results at a UK tertiary hospital. J Obstet Gynaecol. 2004;24:434-40.
5. Park JY, Park SK, Kim DY, et al. The impact of tumor morcellation during surgery on the prognosis of patients with apparently early uterine leiomyosarcoma. Gynecol Oncol. 2011;122:255-9.
6. RCOG. (2019). Morcellation for abdominal or laparoscopic myomectomy or hysterectomy. [online] Available from https://www.rcog.org.uk/guidance/browse-all-guidance/consent-advice/morcellation-for-abdominal-or-laparoscopic-myomectomy-or-hysterectomy-consent-advice-no-13/ [Last accessed November, 2024].
7. Topcu EG, McClenahan P, Pule K, et al. FIGO best practice guidance in surgical consent. Intl J Gynecol Obstetr. 2023;163(3):795-812.
8. Unnecessary Hysterectomies. Dr Narendra Gupta vs Union of India. Writ Petition (Civil) No 131 of 2013; Aril 5, 2023. pp. 57-62.
9. US FDA. (2023). Laparoscopic Power Morcellators. [online] Available from https://www.fda.gov/medical-devices/surgery-devices/laparoscopic-power-morcellators [Last accessed November, 2024].
10. Uterine Morcellation for Presumed Leiomyomas: ACOG Committee Opinion, Number 822. Obstet Gynecol. 2021;137(3):e63-e74.
11. Viswanathan M, Hartmann K, McKoy N, et al. Management of uterine fibroids: an update of the evidence. Evid Rep Technol Assess (Full Rep). 2007;154:1-122.
12. Yuk JS, Kim M. Incidence rates of myomectomy related mortality and venous thromboembolism in South Korea: a population based study. Front Med (Lausanne). 2022;9:849660.